APPLIED
VETERINARY GYNAECOLOGY
AND OBSTETRICS

Dr Pradeep Kumar MVSc, PhD (pursuing)
Division of Animal Reproduction
Indian Veterinary Research Institute
Izatnagar, Bareilly (UP)

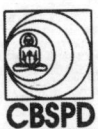

CBSPD

CBS Publishers & Distributors Pvt Ltd

New Delhi • Bengaluru • Chennai • Kochi • Kolkata • Lucknow • Mumbai
Hyderabad • Jharkhand • Nagpur • Patna • Pune • Uttarakhand

APPLIED VETERINARY GYNAECOLOGY AND OBSTETRICS

ISBN: 978-81-239-2785-5

Copyright © Publisher

First CBS Reprint: 2015
Reprint: 2016, 2017, 2020, 2022, 2023 2024

Published by **Satish Kumar Jain** and produced by **Varun Jain** for

CBS Publishers & Distributors Pvt Ltd
4819/XI Prahlad Street, 24 Ansari Road, Daryaganj, New Delhi 110 002, India.
Ph: 011-23289259, 23266861, 23266867
Fax: 011-23243014
Website: www.cbspd.com
e-mail: delhi@cbspd.com;
cbspubs@airtelmail.in.

Corporate Office: 204 FIE, Industrial Area, Patparganj, Delhi 110 092
Ph: 011-4934 4934
Fax: 011-4934 4935
e-mail: publishing@cbspd.com; publicity@cbspd.com

Branches

• **Bengaluru:** Seema House 2975, 17th Cross, KR Road, Banasankari 2nd Stage, Bengaluru 560 070, Karnataka, India
Ph: +91-80-26771678/79   Fax: +91-80-26771680   e-mail: bangalore@cbspd.com
• **Chennai:** 7, Subbaraya Street, Shenoy Nagar, Chennai 600 030, Tamil Nadu, India
Ph: +91-44-26680620, 26681266   Fax: +91-44-42032115   e-mail: chennai@cbspd.com
• **Kochi:** 42/1325, 1326, Power House Road, Opp KSEB, Power House, Ernakulam Kochi 682 018, Kerala, India
Ph: +91-484-4059061-65,67   Fax: +91-484-4059065   e-mail: kochi@cbspd.com
• **Kolkata:** 147, Hind Ceramics Compound, 1st Floor, Nilgunj Road, Belghoria, Kolkata-700056, West Bengal, India
Ph: +033-25633055, 033-25633056   e-mail: kolkata@cbspd.com
• **Lucknow:** Basement, Khushnuma Complex, 7 Meerabai Marg (Behind Jawahar Bhawan),Lucknow-226001, UP, India
Ph: +0522-4000032   e-mail: tiwari.lucknow@cbspd.com
• **Mumbai:** PWD Shed, Gala no 25/26, Ramchandra Bhatt Marg, Next to JJ Hospital Gate no. 2, Opp. Union Bank of India, Noorbaug, Mumbai-400009, Maharashtra, India
Ph: 022-66661880/89   e-mail: mumbai@cbspd.com

Representatives

• Hyderabad   0-9885175004   • Jharkhand   0-9811541605   • Nagpur   0-9421945513
• Patna   0-9334159340   • Pune   0-9623451994   • Uttarakhand   0-9716462459

Printed at   Glorious Printer, Dilshad Garden, Delhi

Perfection is accomplished not by doing extraordinary things, but by doing ordinary things extraordinarily well.

Dedicated
to
my beloved centenarian grandfather

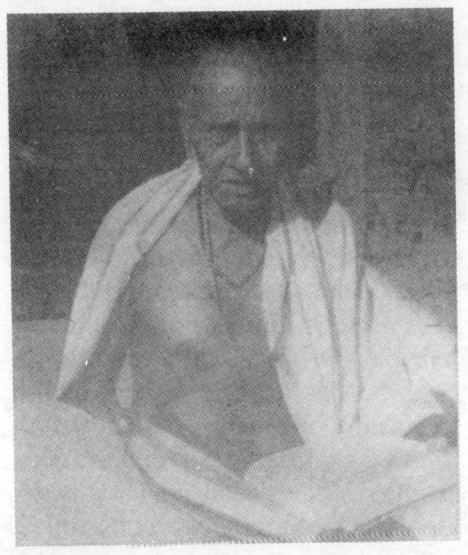

Shri Babujan Prasad
(12.06.1906 - till date)

whose blessings have brought me here upto...

PREFACE

This book has been written for the purpose to cover the practical and clinical aspects of Veterinary Gynaecology and Obstetrics. The author has tried to prepare this book in a unique manner. The matter has been presented in a very simple language and lucrative manner so that one can read this book in one breath. In many books, very exhaustive and huge informations are given but these are very boring task to read for undergraduate students and clinicians. The aim of the book is to tell a scientific and technically sound precise story instead of presenting a data base encyclopaedia on the subject. Therefore the materials has been arranged accordingly and the supplementary informations or more detailed explanations are given in the boxes which can be consulted at once or return to after the principal points have been grasped. For increasing the interest and to give the information of new advances in the field of Veterinary Gynaecology, the author has made his every possible effort. For this, 'Interesting Facts', 'Clinical Pointers', 'Do you know?' 'Points to Remember' etc. have been incorporated in the boxes in between the matter. My main motto in compiling information in this book is to provide relevant information in a simple and interesting way so that matter should not appear difficult to understand by an average undergraduate students. A number of illustrations and photographs have been included to make each chapter meaningful. At the end of each chapter, 'observations' and 'exercise' have been given which will help a clinician in testing his/her acquired knowledge and a student in preparing for examinations and viva-voce. It is hoped that this style of writing will encourage the use of this book for the final year B.V.Sc & A.H., students and Veterinary clinicians.

This book also cover clinical cases of cattle and buffalo in an interesting way with new concepts. Wherever it becomes necessary to point out the old concepts of treatment, I did and highlighted the new concepts of treatments. Thus this book gives an information about latest trend of treatments and explain the disadvantages of adopting old trend of treatments.

In this book, various interesting and clinically important chapters have been included which are generally not given in the text books available in the market. For example, pregnancy diagnosis in small ruminants by 'recto-abdominal palpation', early pregnancy diagnosis in cattle by 'milk ejection test' etc. These are very-very simple and reliable techniques for diagnosis of pregnancy. Generally pregnancy diagnosis in small ruminants requires X-ray and ultrasound because only abdominal palpation is not confirmatory diagnosis. However, use of these sophisticated methods are not feasible in the field conditions, whereas 'recto-abdominal palpation technique' gives 90-100 % accuracy without use of any sophisticated instrument. Likewise the author has tried to give as many such informations which can be applied in Indian field conditions.

Therefore author thinks that this book is a readymade matter on Veterinary Gynaecology and Obstetrics for final year undergraduate students of B.V.Sc. & A.H., field veterinarians and academicians. This book is also useful for various competitive examinations and interviews.

This book has been divided into three parts. In the part I from chapter 1 to 17 are designed to help the final year students, beginners and clinicians to understand the anatomy and physiology of reproduction, gynaecological examinations and their applications to diagnose the clinical problems.

In part II, chapters 18 to 28 emphasize the application of basic concepts of obstetrical cases and their management. In this part, author has tried to explain the basic principles of obstetrics, which are generally over-looked in most of the books available in the market. For example 'how to apply rope on the legs and head of foetus', 'how to prevent the inner wall of uterus and birth canal from the teeth and hooves of the foetus', 'what should be the direction for traction of rope in different stages' etc. Separate obstetrical cases, their incidences, causes and treatments have not been discussed in detail. Foetotomy and caesarean section have been described in detail.

In part III, chapters 29 to 46 have been devoted to the therapeutic management of gynaecological problems. This part describes some of the problems that are commonly encountered in the field. The aim of writing this part is to at least provide a coherent overall therapy guide, create a stimulus and direction for greater in-depth study on particular chapter, and contribute a useful compilation of existing practical therapeutic knowledge for the veterinary undergraduates, clinicians and academicians. Antimicrobial agents are the most frequently used and misused drugs in veterinary practice. A rational approach to antimicrobial therapy entails choosing the proper drug to be administered to the particular animals after considerations of potential benefits and risks. Prerequisites to rational therapy include a diagnosis, understanding of the pathophysiology of the disease and pharmacology of the drug and the establishment of therapeutic objectives. It is the purpose of this part to describe an approach to rational treatment of infections, which cause infertility in cattle and buffaloes. Part III also includes effect of homoeopathic medicines on the female genital tract. Hahnemann (1814) advocated their use in animals and so Veterinary Homoeopathy has a long tradition.

At the end of this book, 'Glossary' and 'Appendix' have been given which will help the veterinary graduates in preparing for various competitive examinations, viva-voce examinations and interviews because these have been collected and arranged in a very lucid manner.

The author encourages constructive comments and valuable suggestions, addition, alteration and correction for any typing error for improving this book in the next edition.

PRADEEP KUMAR

ACKNOWLEDGEMENTS

"Timely help albeit small will ever be greater than the universe.

I would like to thank all known and unknown hands who directly or indirectly gave their valuable contributions in gestation and birth of this book.

In preparing this book, I have been greatly aided by suggestions received from many scientists including **Dr. M.H. Akhtar, Dr. M.R. Ansari, Dr. R.P. Pandey, Dr. G.P. Roy, Dr. A.P. Singh** and **Dr. C. Singh.**

"One who directs the path of progress is angelic." Words are inadequate to express my deep sense of indebtedness to **Dr. G.P. Roy,** for instilling in me a spirit of hope, struggle, determination and affection.

I would like to express my sincere gratitude and thanks to **Dr. Jitendra Kumar Singh** for giving ideas to the use of homoeopathic drugs in bovines.

I am extremely delighted in extending my thanks to **Dr. Rahul Arya, Dr. Neeraj Srivastava, Dr. V.K. Bharti** and **Dr. Braj Bhushan Bachchoo** for their constant encouragement and helping in proof-reading of the manuscript.

My friends and seniors **Dr. Sanjay, Dr. Praveen, Dr. Shantanu, Dr. Nirbhay, Dr. Sunil, Dr. Asthana, Dr. Nishant, Dr. Nirala, Dr. Ajeet, Dr. Kaushal, Dr. Mithilesh, Dr. Dheeraj, Dr. Jeevan, Dr. Zeyaul** and many others deserve sincere thanks for their moral support and valuable suggestions during writing of this book.

"Where emotions are involved, words cease to exist". I admit my inability to put into words, the depth of gratitude and respect. I owe a lot to my parents for the sacrifices made by them at the cost of their comfort and happiness to bring me up to this stage.

Last but not the least, I thank the Almighty for blessing me with indomitable will-power, courage, strength and stamina to accomplish this arduous task.

CONTENTS

Preface

Acknowledgements

PART – I : GYNAECOLOGICAL EXAMINATIONS

PART – II : OBSTETRICS

PART – I

GYNAECOLOGICAL EXAMINATIONS

Special Features :

- Keys or indications used during prescription writing
- Back – pressure test
- Pregnancy diagnosis in small ruminants by 'Recto-abdominal Technique' and 'Mammary Secretion Test'
- Pregnancy diagnosis of cattle by 'Seed Bio-assay Method' and 'Milk-Ejection Test Method'
- TET
- Milk allergy

Chapter 1

Study of Female Genitalia in Slaughter House Specimens

OBJECTIVES :

To know the normal shape and size of different genital organs of different species which help in differentiating the normal and pathological specimens.

MATERIALS REQUIRED :

Preserved or fresh female genital organs of different species, tray, scissors, forceps, BP handle & blade, Scales, Vernier's Calliper, Hand gloves, weight box and balance.

METHOD :

- Place the numbers of genitalia in normal position in a tray.
- Examine all the genitalia by gloved hands only.
- Dilate the vulva with the help of forceps and observe the external urethral orifice and suburethral diverticulum.
- Differentiate the **external urethral orifice** and **suburethral diverticulum** by passing the A.I. gun. AI gun passes into external urethral opening and ultimately goes to urinary bladder while in suburethral diverticulum, AI gun could not be passed.
- Hold the cervix (hard structure) between the index and middle finger of left hand, and with the help of the thumb, palpate the external os of cervix.
- With the help of index, middle finger and thumb, palpate the whole external surface of the cervix to know whether it is hard/ firm or flaccid.
- Palpate body of the uterus.
- Palpate whole surface of the left horn as well as right horn with the help of fingers.

3

- Palpate the fallopian tubes by stretching the mesosalpinx.
- Catch the ovary and fix between the index and middle finger and palpate its whole surface with the help of thumb for the presence of follicles (**elevated soft fluid filled structure**) corpus luteum (**elevated hard structure**) and corpus albicans.
- Dissect the cervix with the help of BP blade and scissors longitudinally and observe the annular rings.
- Dissect the body of uterus and horns and observe the partition between two horns.
- Count the number of caruncles and its arrangement in ruminant.

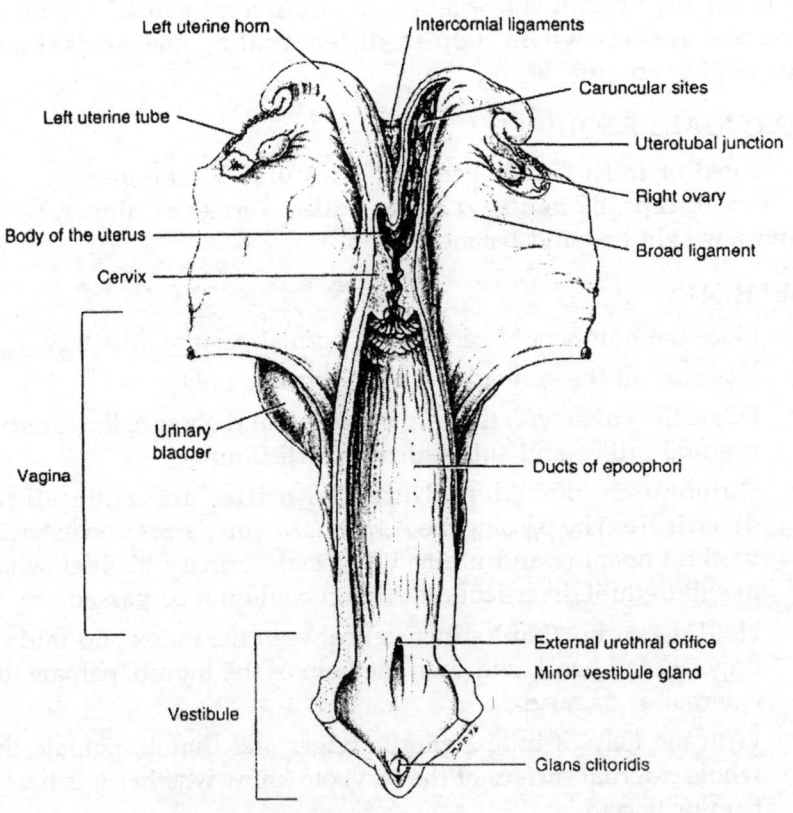

Fig. 1.1 : The reproductive tract of a cow, opened dorsally through the caudal half of the right horn of the uterus.

INTERESTING FACTS

- Increasing age and parity result in larger size of the cervix.
- The true bifurcation of horns is found at the junction of horns with the body of uterus while false bifurcation is located further forward at the site where both horns are connected by two intercornual ligaments.
- The ventral intercornual ligament is stronger than the dorsal intercornual ligament.
- Cows have larger ovaries than heifers.
- Ovaries, which do not contain functional structures such as the corpora lutea and Graafian follicles, are almond shaped. Presence of developed corpora lutea in the ovary results in marked distorsion in its shape.
- A 'yellow' corpus luteum is either developing or regressing.
- Wrinkles on vulva are present in the cows while they are absent in buffaloes.
- Buffalo vagina is shorter as compared to that of cow.

Measure the length and diameter of all parts of genitalia with the help of measuring scale and thread as mentioned below and make a comparison among different genitallia and with that of normal.

(a) Vulva :

Length - From ventral commissure to external urethral opening.

Height - Distance between ventral and dorsal commissure.

(b) Vagina :

Length - Distance between external urethral opening and fornix.

(c) Cervix :

Length - From external os to internal os.

Width - External diameter of middle portion.

Thickness - Actual thickness of the wall.

Circumference - Measure externally

(d) Uterine horns :

Length - From internal bifurcation to apex. i.e. ovarian end.

Thickness - Actual thickness of the wall.

Circumference - Measure externally

(e) Fallopian tubes :

Length - From uterine extremity to infundibulum.

Thickness - Actual thickness of the wall.

Circumference - Measure externally.

(f) Ovary :

Length - From anterior to posterior extremity.

Width - Greatest diameter between lateral and medial borders.

Thickness - From attached border to free border.

Weight - Cut the ovary and take the weight on balance.

Various phases of corpora lutea related to various stages of estrous cycle

Finding	Stage of estrous cycle (days)
Ovulation depression	1-2 days
Soft developing CL not exceeding 1 cm in diameter	2-3 days
Soft developing CL 1-2 cm in diameter	3-5 days
Soft developing CL more than 2 cm in diameter	5-7 days
Fully developed CL	8-17 days
Firm CL 1-2 cm in diameter	18-20 days
Hard CL less than 1 cm. in diameter	Estrus to middle of the subsequent cycle.

OBSERVATIONS :

Vulva

Length (cm) ....

Height (cm) ....

Vagina

Length (cm) ....

Cervix

Length (cm) ....

Width (cm) ....

	Left	Right
Thickness (cm)	....	
Uterine body		
Length (cm)	....	
Thickness (cm)	....	
Uterine horns		
Length (cm)	....	....
Thickness (cm)	....	....
Circumference (cm)	....	....
Fallopian tubes		
Length (cm)	....	....
Thickness (mm)	....	....
Circumference (cm)	....	....
Ovary		
Length (cm)	....	....
Width (cm)	....	....
Thickness (cm)	....	....
Follicles	*Present/Absent*	*Present/Absent*
Corpus luteum	....	....
Size of projected portion of CL		
Height (mm)	....	....
Width (mm)	....	....

EXERCISE :

1. How the caruncles remain arranged in uterine horns ?

Ans. -

2. What is the total number of caruncles in different species ?

Ans. -

3. What is the colour of mature corpus luteum in cow ?

Ans. -

4. What is the colour of corpus albicans in cow ?

Ans. -

5. During PM examination, how & what conclusion can be made by examining the ovary regarding the number of pregnancy/ parity carried out by that cow in her life ?

Ans. -

6. In which animal (Zebu cattle/Exotic cattle) vulvar lips are bigger and more prominent ?

Ans. -

7. In which animal (Zebu cattle/Exotic cattle) cervix is two to three times bigger than other?

Ans. -

8. The ovaries of which animal (Zebu cattle/Exotic cattle) are larger ?

Ans. -

9. In which animal (Zebu cattle/Exotic cattle), assessment of corpus luteum by rectal palpation is comparatively difficult & why ?

Ans. –

❊ ❊ ❊ ❊ ❊

> The opportunity for doing mischief is found a hundred times a day and of doing good, once a year.   - Voltaire.

Chapter 2

Comparative Anatomy of Reproductive Tracts

The organs of female genital system are ovaries, oviducts, uterus, vagina and vulva(see table)

Ovaries :

These are two oval bodies one on each side, situated slightly above to the middle of the pelvic inlet and are attached to the broad ligament by a fold of peritoneum called **mesovarium**. The size of ovary is highly variable from animal to animal. The average length of ovary of cow is 2-3 cm; width is 2cm. and thickness is 1cm. The ovaries of ewe and doe are less than half the size of those of a cow while the ovaries of mare are two to three times larger than those of a cow. The ovaries of the sow are slightly larger than those found in the ewe.

Each ovary has **two borders, two surfaces** and **two ends**. The surfaces (lateral and medial) are convex and irregular in appearance. The ovary is attached with the mesovarium by one border and the free border is convex.

INTERESTING FACTS
• For unknown reasons, the two ovaries do not function equally in most domestic species.
• According to an opinion the blood supply to an ovary might influence the amount of gonadtropins reaching the ovary which in turn command the ovarian function.
• In ruminants, presence of rumen in left side perhaps restricts the blood supply to the left ovary. Therefore, left ovary is less active than the right ovary.
• In the ewe, 55 to 60% of ova come from the right ovary and in the cow, 60-65% of the ova come from the right ovary.
• In the sow, left ovary is most active, 55 to 60% of the ova come from the left ovary.
• The mare is also a left ovulator with approximately 60% of the ova come from the left ovary.

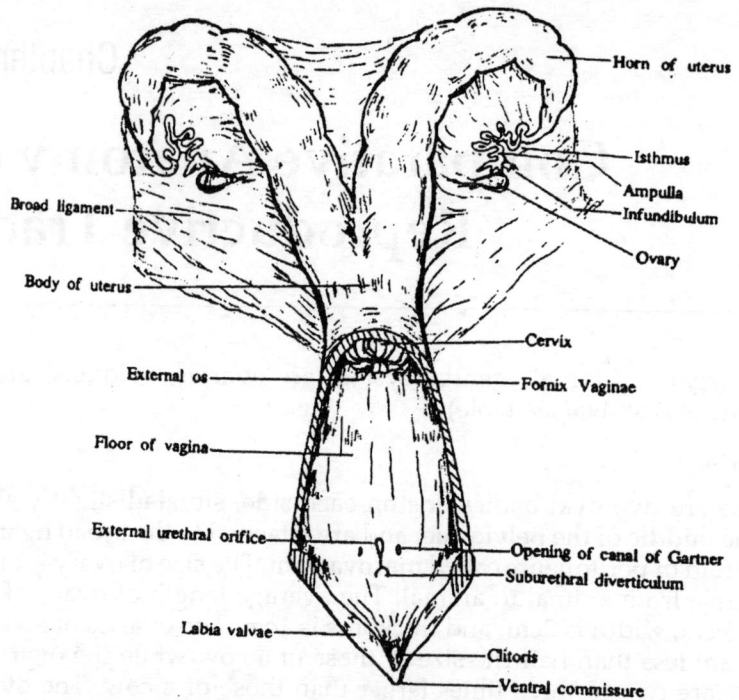

Fig. 2.1 : Female genitalia of a cow. (Courtesy of Ghosh, R.K. 1995. Primary Veterinary Anatomy. Current Book International)

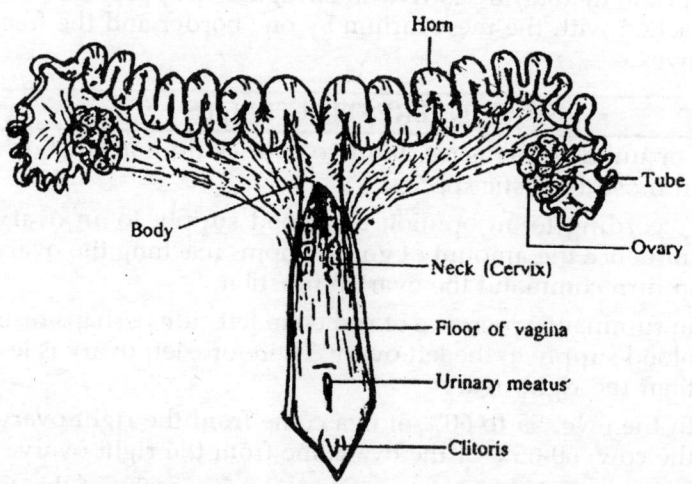

Fig. 2.2 : Genitalia of a sow (Roof of vagina and vulva removed). (Courtesy of Ghosh, R.K. 1995. Primary Veterinary Anatomy. Current Book International)

Different shapes of the ovaries are described in different species :

Cow, She buffalo, ewe & doe -   Almond-shaped

Mare -   Bean-shaped (kidney-shaped)

Sow -   Resembling cluster of grapes (berry-shaped)

Function :

● Oogenesis (Exocrine)

● Secretes oestrogen, progesterone, oxytocin · and relaxin (Endocrine).

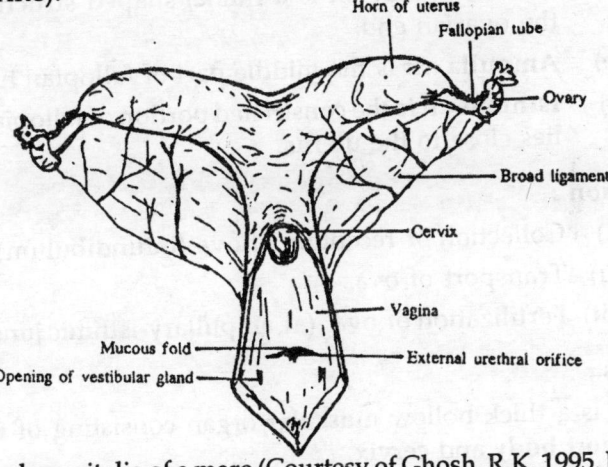

Fig. 2.3 : Female genitalia of a mare (Courtesy of Ghosh, R.K. 1995. Primary Veterinary Anatomy. Current Book International)

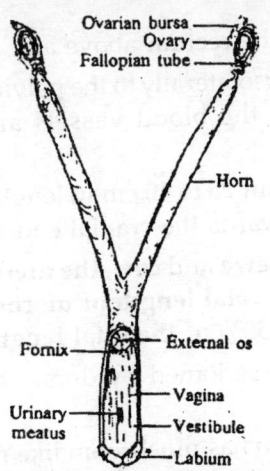

Fig. 2.4 : Female genitalia of a bitch (Courtesy of Ghosh, R.K. 1995. Primary Veterinary Anatomy. Current Book International)

Uterine tubes :

- The uterine tubes are also called **oviducts or fallopian tubes or salpinges.**
- These are paired and convoluted tubes extending from ovaries to uterus.
- Each has a length of about 20-30 cm. and diameter about 2 to 3 mm. in most farm species.
- Each fallopian tube is divided into three parts :
  a) **Infundibulum** : It is a funnel-shaped structure located at the ovarian end.
  b) **Ampulla** : It is the middle part of fallopian tube.
  c) **Isthmus** : It is the constricted portion of fallopian tube which lies close to the uterus.

Function :

(i) Collection or reception of ova (infundibulum).
(ii) Transport of ova.
(iii) Fertilization of ova (at ampullary-isthmic junction).

Uterus :

- It is a thick hollow muscular organ consisting of **two horns, a short body** and **cervix.**
- It is normally situated in the pelvic cavity in non-pregnant females.
- It is related to the rectum above and urinary bladder below.
- It is attached dorsolaterally to the pelvic cavity by **broad ligament** through which the blood vessels and nerves passes, called **mesometrium.**
- Each horn is about 25 to 40 cm in length and 1.5 to 5 cm in width but tapering towards the cranial end (cow).
- **In the sow, doe, ewe and cow, the uterine horns comprise about 80 to 90% of the total length of uterus while in the mare, they comprise about 50% of the total length of uterus.**
- Both the horns are joined by dorsal and ventral **intercornual ligaments.**
- The endometrium has mushroom like non-glandular projections called **caruncles**(ruminants)
- These caruncles are arranged in four rows viz. two dorsal rows and two ventral rows.

- The inter-caruncular spaces contain many blood vessels and uterine glands.
- These caruncles are convex in shape and about 70-120 in number in cow.

Type of uterus

Four basic types of uteri are found in animals :

- **Simple uterus :** When a uterus has a pear-shaped body with no uterine horns, it is called simple uterus. eg., human being and other primates (Fig. 2.7).
- **Bicornuate uterus :** When a uterus has a small uterine body and two long uterine horns, it is called bicornuate uterus. eg., sow, bitch, queen, cow, ewe and doe (Fig. 2.5).
- **Bipartite uterus :** When a uterus has a prominent uterine body and two uterine horns that are not as long and distinct as in bicornuate type, is called bipartite uterus. eg., mare (Fig 2.6).
- **Duplex uterus :** When a uterus has two uterine horns each with a separate cervical canal which opens into vagina, it is called duplex uterus. eg., rat, rabbit, guinea pig and other small animals (Fig. 2.7).

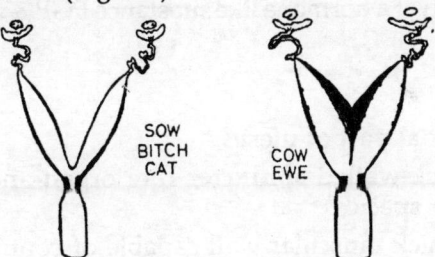

Fig. 2.5 : Bicornuate Uterus

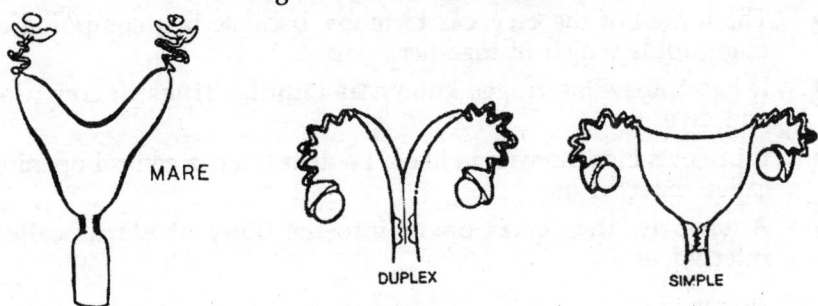

Fig. 2.6 : Bipartite Uterus   Fig. 2.7 : Duplex and Simple Uterus

INTERESTING FACT
Fusion of the uterine horns of the cow, doe and ewe near the uterine body give the impression of a larger uterine body due to false birfurcation than actually exists. Therefore some authors classified these uteri as bipartite uterus.

Blood supply

- **Utero-ovarian artery** - Fallopian tubes and anterior part of uterine horns.

- **Middle uterine artery** – Posterior part of horns and anterior part of body of uterus.

- **Caudal uterine artery** - Posterior part of body of uterus and anterior part of vagina.

Function :

- Transport of sperm towards the fallopian tubes.

- Implantation of zygote.

- Nourishment of embryo during early stage by secreting **uterine milk**.

- Protection of foetus.

- Production of a hormone like substance $PGF_2\alpha$ which has luteolytic effect.

Cervix :

- It is a caudal part of uterus.

- It is a thick-walled **sphincter like** organ and 5-10 cm long in most farm species.

- It has a thick muscular wall capable of contracting to close the passage or capable of relaxing at oestrus or parturition time.

- The lumen of the cervix is tortuous, because it is composed of many folds which fit together.

- It has transverse ridges known as **annular rings** in cow, doe and ewe.

- It projects into the vagina like a knob and has a central opening called **external os.**

- Anteriorly, the cervix opens into the body of uterus called **internal os.**

Function :

- It acts as **sperm reservoir.**

14

- It helps in sperm transport.
- It helps in selection of viable sperm thus preventing the transport of non-viable and defective sperm (**filtration of sperm**).
- It secretes mucus during oestrus period.
- It acts as a barrier against ascending type of infections.
- It forms cervical seal during gestation/pregnancy.

Vagina :

- The vagina is a highly **elastic musculo-membranous tube** located within the pelvis above the urinary bladder and below the rectum.
- It is cranially attached to the uterus and caudaly to the vulva.
- It is about **25-30 cm.** long in **cow and mare** and **10-15 cm long** in **sow, doe and ewe.**
- It serves as a **sheath for the male penis** during copulation.
- The luminal space around the cervix is called **fornix.**
- The external urethral orifice is the **landmark junction of vagina and vulva.** i.e. vagina is extended from the cervix to the external urethral office.
- The cow is unique in possessing an anterior sphincter muscle in addition to the posterior sphincter.
- At the floor of vagina, there are two ducts along the length of the tube between the muscular and mucus layers, called **canals of Gartner** which open on either side of the external urethral opening. These are the **remanants of wolffian (mesonephric) ducts.**

Function :

- It acts as a copulatory organ of females.
- It serves as an excretory duct for the secretion of cervix, endometrium and oviduct.
- It serves as the birth canal during parturition.

Vulva :

- The vulva or external genitalia consist of the **vestibule** and the **labia.**
- The vestibule is that portion of the female duct system which is common to both the **reproductive and urinary systems.**

15

- The vestibule is extended from the **external urethral orifice** to the **exterior.**

- The vestibule is **10-12 cm** in length in the **cow and mare, half that length** in the **sow** and **one-quarter that length** in the ewe and doe.

- The vestibule is **homologous to the penile urethra** in the male.

- **The vestibular glands or Bartholian glands** (two almond shape) located under the mucus membrane in the posterior part of the vestibule, are active during oestrus and secrete a lubricating mucus.

- These glands keep the vulva of the cow moist during oestrus.

- The vestibular glands are **homologous** to the **bulbourethral glands or cowper's gland** of the male.

- A hymen (transverse ridge) is located at the junction of vagina and vestibule which is **well defined** in the **ewe and mare**, but **ill defined** in the **cow and sow.**

- **The labia** consist of the **labia minora** and **labia majora.**

- **The labia minora is homologous** to the **prepuce** in the male and is not prominent in farm animals.

- **The labia majora is homologous** to the **scrotum** in the male – is that portion of the female system which is visible externally.

- In the cow the labia majora is covered with fine hair up to the mucosa.

- The external opening of vulva is in the form of a slit bounded by two labia which meet at upper and lower commissure.

- The **upper commissure** is acute and separated from anus by a short distance.

- The **lower commissure** is elongated and bears a tuft of hairs.

- The clitoris, **homologous** to the **glans penis** in the male, is located in ventral commissure about 1cm inside the labia.

- In the mare during oestrus, frequent contractions of the labia (winking) expose the erected clitoris.

Broad ligament :

- It is formed by double fold of peritonium with some connective tissue and muscle fibres in between them.

- It provides passage of the nerves and vesseis to the uterus.

16

Table : Comparative Anatomy of the Female Genital Organs.

	Cow	Ewe	Sow	Mare	Bitch	Cat
				Animal		
Ovary						
Shape	Almond - shaped	Almond-shaped	Berry-shaped (Cluster of grapes)	Kidney-shaped with ovulation fossa	Oval. Slightly Flattened	Oval. Slightly Flattened
Weight of one ovary (gm)	10-20	3-4	3-10	40-80	1-8	1-3
Mature Graafian follicles						
Diameter (mm)	12-19	5-10	8-12	25-70	2-4	1-2
Ovary which is the more active	Right	Right	Left	Left	--	--
Mature corpus luteum						
Shape	Spheroid or ovoid	Spheroid or ovoid	Spheroid or ovoid	Pear-shaped	Spheroid	Spheroid
Diameter (mm)	20-25	9	10-15	10-25	2-5	1.5-3
Maximum size attained (days from ovulation)	10	7-9	14	14	5-14	5-14
Regression starts (days from ovulation)	14-15	12-14	13	17	--	--
Uterine tube						
Length (cm)	25	15-19	14-30	20-30	4-7	3-5
Uterus						
Type	Bocornuate	Bocornuate	Bocornuate	Bipartite	Bicornuate	Bicornuate
Length of horn (cm)	35-40	10-12	40-110	15-25	10-14	6-10
Length of body (cm)	2-4	1-2	5	15-20	1.4-2	1.5-2
Numbers of caruncles	70-120 caruncles	88-96 caruncles	Slight longitudinal	Conspicuous Longitudinal folds	Longitudinal Folds	Longitudinal Folds
Cervix						
Length (cm)	8-10	4-10	10-23	7-8	1.5-2	1-1.5
Outside diameter (cm)	3-4	2-3	2-3	3.5-4	5-1.5	4-6
Cervical lumen						
Shape	2-5 Annular rings	Annular rings	Corkscrew-like	Conspicuous folds	Irregular	Irregular
Vagina						
Length (cm)	25-30	10-14	10-23	20-35	5-10	--
Hymen	Ill-defined	Well-developed	Ill-defined	Well-developed	Ill-defined	Ill-defined
Vestibule						
Length (cm)	10-12	2.5-3	6-8	10-12	2-5	5-1.5

All data vary with age, breed and parity and one are only estimates.

17

- Different portions of broad ligaments are attached to different structure of female genitalia and have been named accordingly.
  - Mesovarium   -   Ovary
  - Mesosalpinx -   Fallopian tube
  - Mesometrium -   Uterus

EXERCISE :

1. What are the different types of uterus in farm animal ?

Ans. -

2. What do you mean by corpus luteum spurium and corpus luteum verum.

Ans. -

3. What do you mean by ovulation fossa ?

Ans. -

4. Which artery supplies major blood to the uterus ?

Ans. -

5. Do all domestic animals (intact females) ovulate over the entire surface of the ovary ?

Ans. -

6. Is the cervix remain open at all the time ?

Ans.

7. In which species, fornix is absent ?

Ans. –

8. What is the landmark junction of vagina and vulva ?

Ans. -

9. What is the peculiarity of cow's vagina ?

Ans. –

10. What is the "canal of Gartner" ?

Ans. –

11. What is the 'glands of Bartholin' and its function ?

Ans. –

12. In which species, clitoris is well developed ?

Ans. -

13. What is difference between bicornuate uterus and bipartite uterus ?

Ans. -

14. Which ovary is more active in cattle and why ?

Ans. –

15. Which ovary is more active in mare and why ?

Ans. -

16. Write the homologous organs of the male
    - Clitoris ....
    - Labia minora ....
    - Labia majora ....
    - Vestibule ....
    - Vestibular gland ....

❋ ❋ ❋ ❋ ❋

Only those who dare to fail greatly can ever achieve greatly.

Chapter 3

Per-rectal Palpation of Female Genital Organs

Per-rectal examination is the only practical diagnostic method permitting direct examination of genital organs of a cow, buffalo and mares. However in small animals genital organs are examined via abdominal palpation.

MATERIALS REQUIRED :

Thin full arm plastic gloves, crate, apron, gumboots, soap, water, towel and lubricant.

PROCEDURE AND PRECAUTIONS :

1. Nails should be properly trimmed and rasped.
2. Finger rings, wrist-watch or *kadas* should be removed to avoid injury to rectal mucosa.
3. Wear protective clothings, gloves and gumboots.
4. Apply lubricant over the glove.
5. Restrain the animal properly in a crate.
6. Hold the tail of animal resting on its back.
7. Clean the perineal and vulval region with water.
8. Lubricate the anal sphincter by putting index finger and dilate it.
9. Now put all fingers with index fingers making a cone shape of the hand and insert it for the examination.
10. Remove the faeces (back-racking) without removing the hand out of the rectum to avoid rectal ballooning by sucking of air in it.
11. If ballooning occurs, reduce it by gentle pinching the rectal floor at its anteriormost folds.

12. Do not examine during peristaltic wave of rectum and/or when the animal is straining or tenesmus is present.

13. Avoid force during examination.

14. Insert hand up to pelvic brim.

15. Locate the cervix as a firm tubular structure approximately 25-35 cm from the anal sphincter.

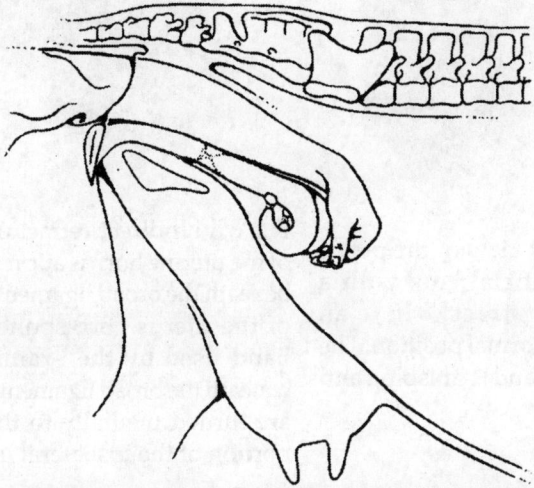

Fig. 3.1 : Palpation of the uterus (diagrammatic) which can be scooped up by the hand as it lies in the abdominal cavity.

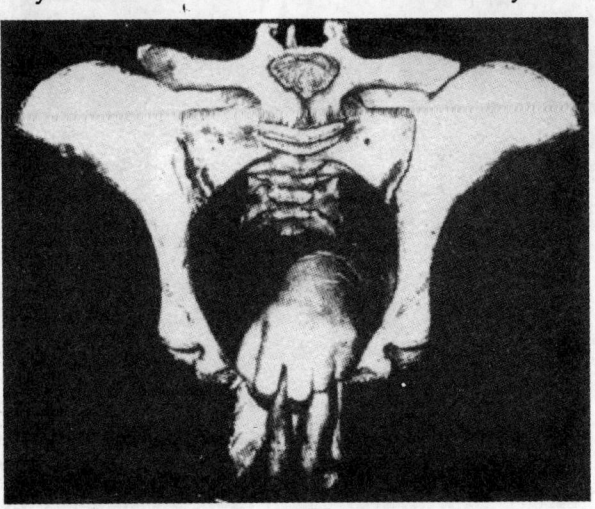

Fig. 3.2 : Retraction of a uterus lying well within the abdominal cavity by means of the false bifurcation.

21

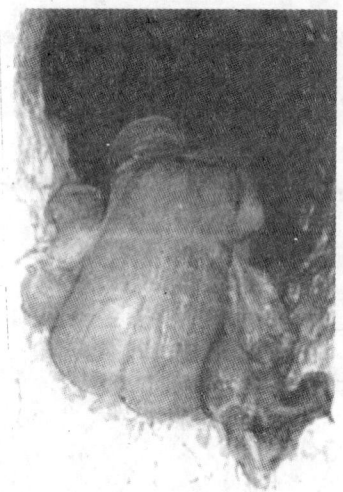

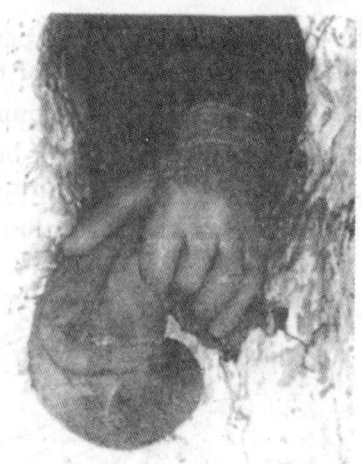

Fig. 3.3 : Cranial view of the pelvic inlet of an artificial cow with a reproductive tract in an approximately normal position. The examiner's left hand is grasping and raising the cervix.

Fig. 3.4 : Indirect retraction. The end of the uterine horn is approached from beneath the broad ligament on the side of the uterus corresponding to the hand used by the examiner. From beneath the broad ligament, the fingers are turned medially to find the free portion of the ipsilateral horn.

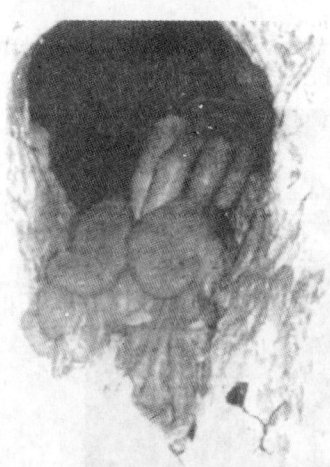

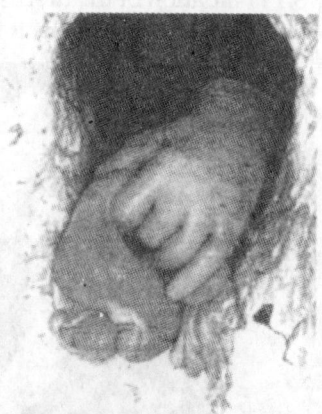

Fig. 3.5 : Direct retraction may be accomplished if the ventral intercornual ligament is directly accessible to raise and uncoil the tract.

Fig. 3.6 : Indirect retraction. The uterine horn is cradled in the fingers and palpated, progressing caudally until the index finger meets the intercornual ligament.

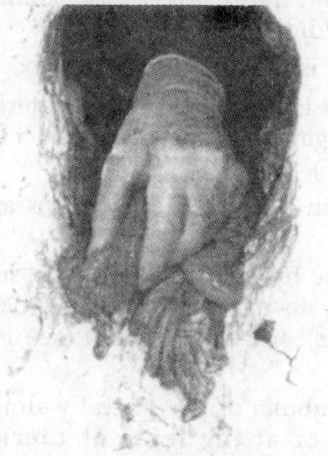

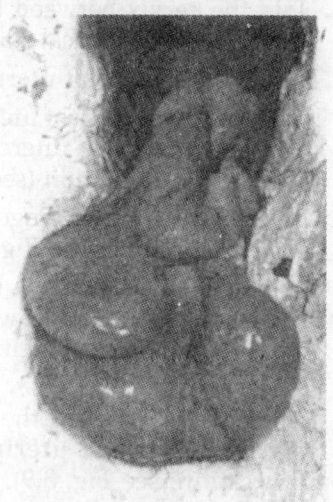

Fig. 3.7 : Palpation of the free portion of the uterine horn opposite the hand of the examiner.

Fig. 3.8 : A pregnancy of approximately 75 days'. The pregnant right horn rests against the prepubic tendon.

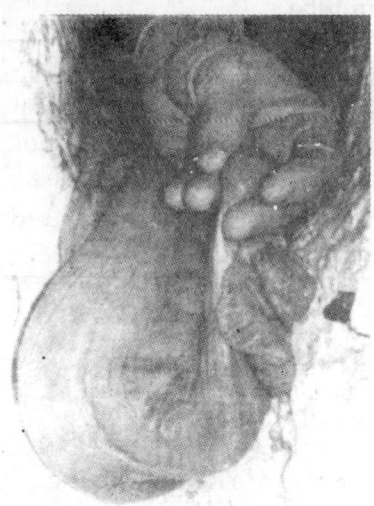

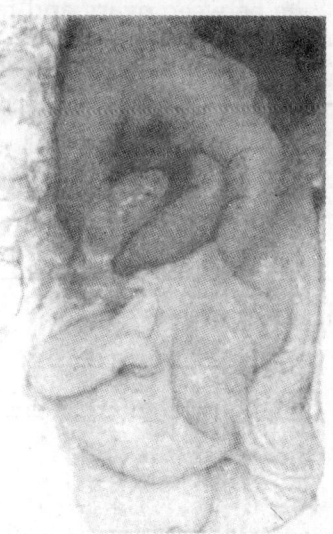

Fig. 3.9 : Palpation of the left ovary fixed between the fingers and palpated with the thumb.

Fig. 3.10 : The right ovary of a cow, demonstrating a corpus luteum. (Courtesy of Wolfe, F.D. and Moll, H.D. 1999. Large Animal Urogenital Surgery for all figures of this chapter.)

16. Hold the cervix between thumb and index finger and examine its physio-pathological status including external os.

17. Examine the body of uterus which is in continuity of cervix.

18. Anterior to the body of uterus, there is false bifurcation of uterine horns attached with intercornual ligament. If needed, retract the organ for examination (see Fig. 3.5)

19. Put middle or index finger between the two uterine horns and locate the intercornual ligament.

20. Palpate both the uterine horns one by one by digital pressure from base to tip to know the physio- pathological conditions like its symmetry, tonicity and for content (like pus) (see Fig. 3.5).

21. Ovaries are located by the side of tubular organ- laterally almost near to the tip of uterine horn or **at the level of uterine bifurcation** (see Fig. 3.9).

22. Hold the ovary between middle and index finger and palpate by thumb for presence or absence of functional structure over the ovary (see Figs 3.9 & 3.10).

23. Fallopian tubes are normally not palpable except in pathological condition. However, ovarian bursa may be examined by rotating the two (middle and index) fingers on the broad ligament at the site between ovary and fallopian tube.

Important points to remember :
• The empty uterus usually contracts in response to palpation.
• Since reflex contractions of the uterus impede palpation, so it should be palpated before attending to the ovaries.
• The diameter of the uterine horns can be measured by comparison with finger's diameter.

Palpation of cervix :

Finding		Diagnosis
• Symmetrical enlargement	-	Diffuse inflammation
	-	Recent calving
	-	Abortion
• Symmetrical enlargement with pain	-	Septic condition
• Asymmetrical enlargement	-	Abscess
	-	Injury
	-	Scar

- External os is large and show step like appearance – Second degree cervicitis
- External os is large and show clear step like protrusion – Third degree cervicitis

Palpation of uterus :

Commonly used terms for characterizing uterine tone and condition of uterine tissue :

- **Estrus tone** – A turgid, **contracted uterus** that is often curled during palpation.
- **Dioestrus (normal)** – A relaxed muscular uterus.
- **Oedematous** – Somewhat turgid uterus but **without muscular contraction;** may be palpable for a few days after oestrus.
- **Flaccid** – A flexible, soft, usually thin-walled uterus that **does not contract** in response to palpation.
- **Thickened (doughy)** – A pathological condition, indicating thickning of the endometrium and myometrium.
- **Fluctuant** – Uterus with intraluminal fluid.
- **Firmness** – Chronic inflammation or neoplasia.
- **Longitudinal folds** – Involuting uterus.

The following keys or indications can be used to record the results of palpation of the uterus in prescription.

Key		Size of uterus
U I	–	Uterus can be gathered up within the hand; horns about the thickness of a finger.
U II	–	As above, but the horns about the thickness of **two fingers.**
U III	–	As above, but the horns about the thickness of **3 or 4 fingers.**
U IV	–	It is thicker than **human arm** and greater curvature of the horns is still within reach.
U V	–	Uterus cannot quite be covered by the hand and part of the greater curvature of the horns is out of reach.
U VI	–	Uterus is much bigger than the span of a hand and the greater curvature is quite distinctly out of reach.

Symmetry of uterus :

Key		Symmetry of uterus
S	-	Both horns of the same size (symmetrical)
As	-	The horns are of different size (asymmetrical)
As+++	-	The right horn is much bigger than the left.
+As	-	The left horn is somewhat longer than the right.

Consistency and contractibility of uterus :

Key :

C I	-	Uterus slack and not very contractile.
C II	-	Moderate contractibility.
C III	-	Strong contractibility.

Palpation of ovary :

- Vesicles can be felt on the bovine ovary at all stages of the reproductive cycle.

- A vesicle with a thin wall, 1.5 cm. in diameter (sometimes up to 2.5 cm. diameter) and accompanied by pronounced contractibility of the uterus will be mature Graafian follicle of oestrus.

- Mature Graafian follicle is frequently found towards the end of first half of the oestrous cycle *i.e.* first wave of follicle formation. At this stage either ovary also bears large corpus luteum, which is not usually present during oestrus.

- A cavity up to 1cm deep on the surface of the ovary marks the site of ovulation (providing there are also external and internal signs of recent oestrus).

- Between the 2nd and 5th (6th) days of the cycle, there are neither vesicles nor solid structures (corpus luteum). This appearance can be confused with an inactive ovary. For this, re-examine the animal few days later.

- A small, soft, periodic corpus luteum can be felt from the 5th day of the cycle onwards.

- Most CL have a **papilla or crown like projection or neck** above the surface of the ovary.

- **Corpus albicans** are small and very firm structure which can be differentiated from fluctuating structure of Graafian follicles.

Results of ovarian palpation can be recorded according to the following keys or indications in the prescription.

- **Shape of the ovary-** can be shown in a drawing, in which a **vesicle** is depicted as **empty**, while a **corpus luteum** is **shaded**.
- **Size of ovary :**

Key		Size
Pe	=	Pea
B	=	Bean
Ha	=	Hazel nut
Pi	=	Pigeon's egg
W	=	Walnut
He	=	Hen's egg
D	=	Duck's egg
G	=	Goose's egg

- **The abbreviations employed for various structures of ovary.**

LO	=	Left ovary
RO	=	Right ovary
DF	=	Developing follicle
AF	=	Atretic follicle
TF	=	Tense follicle
SF	=	Soft follicle
OVD	=	Ovulatory depression
SDCL	=	Soft developing corpus luteum
FDCL	=	Fully developed corpus luteum
FCL	=	Firm corpus luteum
HCL	=	Hard corpus luteum
PCL	=	Persistent corpus luteum
CO	=	Cystic ovary
CCL	=	Cystic corpus luteum
LC	=	Luteal cyst
OBA	=	Ovario-bursal adhesions

OBSERVATIONS :

1. Cervix

- Location (pelvic/abdominal) ....
- Condition (normal/inflammed) ....
- External os (open/close) ....
- Length (cm) ....

2. Uterus

- Uterine tone ....
- Condition of uterine tissue ....
- Size ....
- Symmetry ....
- Consistency and contractibility ....
- Abnormality, if any ....

3. Oviduct

- Palpated *Yes/No*

4. Ovary : **Left** **Right**

Size ....

Follicle ....

Corpus luteum ....

Tentative diagnosis : ....

EXERCISE :

1. Why uterus should be palpated before ovary ?

Ans.

2. Why back racking should be done without removing hand from the rectum ?

Ans.

3. Where ovaries are located during per rectal examination ?

Ans.

4. What indicate the longitudinal folds on the uterus ?

Ans.

5. A doctor makes a sketch-diagram and uses abbreviation on a prescription after per rectal examination. What does indicate each sketch-diagram ?

Sketch diagram   **Description**

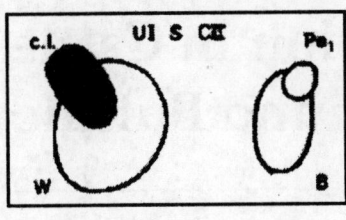
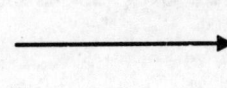

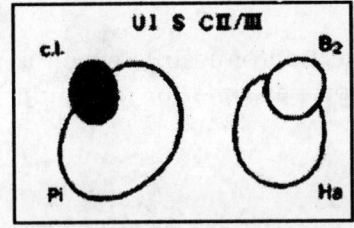
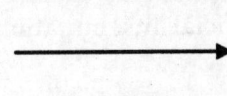

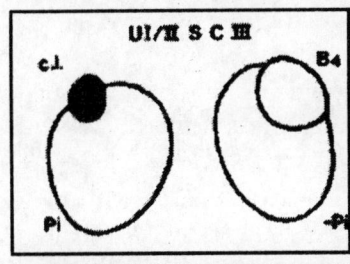
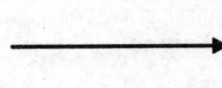

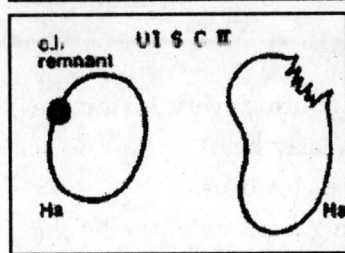
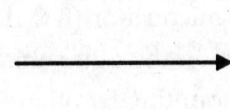

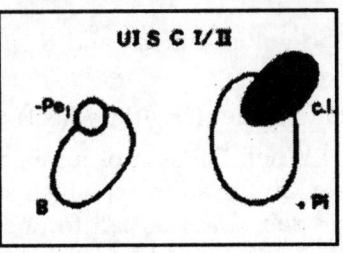
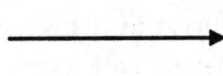

Chapter 4

Oestrus Detection in Cattle and Buffalo

OBJECTIVE :

To know different methods used for detection of oestrus which is essential for artificial insemination at proper time for optimum conception rate.

MATERIALS REQUIRED :

Teaser, trained dogs, glass slide, a pair scissors, arm-sleeves, gumboots, soap, towel etc.

DIFFERENT METHODS :

1) **By behavioural signs :**
   - Restlessness
   - Bellowing frequently
   - Spontaneous sinking of the loin
   - Reduced appetite
   - Fall in milk yield
   - Frequent micturition (few drops of urine every 3-5 minutes)
   - Mounting on the other animals (**early heat**)
   - Accept mounting by other animals (**mid heat**)
   - Mucus discharge flows as a string from vulva to the floor and breaks (**early heat**)
   - Mucus discharge hangs from the vulva to hock and then breaks off (**mid heat**)
   - The mucus string hangs only 25 to 30 cm long (**late heat**)
   - **Loin reflex or Tolerance reflex :** When the skin of lumbar and sacral vertebral region is held, all the animals will sink their back, but the animal in oestrus raises its tail to one

side of the vulvar lips in addition to sinking its back. This is called **loin reflex**. If the animal is not in heat, it raises the tail above vulvar lips, not one side of the vulvar lips (see Fig. 4.1).

- In buffaloes, the skin is kneaded from lumbar region to the base of the tail repeatedly without lapse of time between kneadings and if she is in heat, raises the tail to one side of the vulvar lips. This is called "**Tail Reflex**".

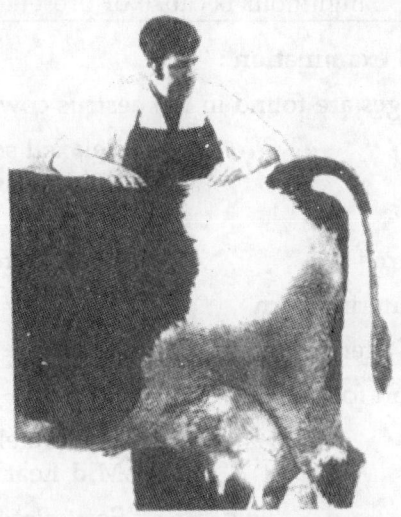

Fig. 4.1 : Tolerance reflex : When the lumbo-sacral region is massaged, the cow in oestrus will sink its back and raise its tail to one side. (Courtesy of Rosenberger, G. 1997. Clincal Examination of Cattle Verlag Paul Parey. Berlin and Hamburg.)

- **Clitoris massage reflex**: When ventral vulvar lips are massaged gently, the animal in heat bends and raises its back repeatedly simultaneously contracts the abdomen with raising the tail to one side of the vulval lips.

Note: Most of the buffaloes get excited on this test. Hence this test should not be performed for the detection of oestrus in buffaloes.

IMPORTANT POINT
The external signs of oestrus which are mentioned above, not necessarily each and every cow show all signs simultaneously. Hence, for confirmation, more or less apparent external signs necessitate to check the genital system by rectal examination and vaginal examination.

Characteristics of mucus discharge :	
Early oestrus	- Clear, thin and copious, flows stringy from vulva to the ground
Mid oestrus	- Clear, less copious and stringy, hangs upto hocks
Late oestrus	- Clear, thick, scanty and non sticky
After ovulation	- Yellowish white
Metoestrus	- Sanguinous because of presence of blood

2. By per-rectal examination :

Following changes are found in the oestrus cow/buffalo

- Cervix — Relaxed so that the **tip of thumb can be inserted into os**
- Tonicity of uterus — Tonic & turgid
- Tubularity of uterine horn — Round or flat
- Consistency of uterine horn — Meaty
- Mature Graafian follicle — Bulged & Firm – **Early heat**

  Moderately flat and soft– **Mid heat**

  Soft – **late heat**
- No evidence of mature corpus luteum

3. By vaginal examination :

Vulval oedema and **disappearance of wrinkles.**

- Entire part of vulval lips light pink - **Early heat**
- Entire vulval lips dark pink - **Mid heat**
- Entire vulval lips cyanotic - **Late heat**

4. By laboratory diagnosis :

Laboratory diagnosis of oestrus requires expensive equipments, the procedure is time consuming and it does not give a clear-cut result in every case. Therefore such methods are unsuitable for routine use. The only laboratory method suitable for use in cattle practice is measurement of the electrical resistance of vaginal mucus. Values less than 40 ohms are characteristics of oestrus.

5. By a teaser bull :

- In a large farm, use of teaser bull for detection of heat is the most reliable and successful method.
- Parading the teaser bull twice daily in the herd.

6. By a trained dog :

Some pheromones are used to communicate information concerned with reproduction called **sex pheromones**. The external genitalia and urine contain these pheromones. When a dog is trained with cow's vaginal fluid, then the dog can detect oestrus cow (87% accuracy). This inter-species detection of pheromones helps in identifying oestrus in a herd where artificial insemination is to be used.

INTERESTING FACTS

DETECTION OF SPLIT OESTRUS :

In split oestrus, the animal show behavioural oestrus twice within a period of 3 to 6 days. The first oestrus is generally non-ovulatory while the second oestrus is ovulatory. It is common in winter.

DETECTION OF MID-CYCLE OESTRUS :

Animals having large follicle and regressed CL on either ovary are considered standing oestrus while those having fully developed CL co-existing with palpable ovarian follicle (10 mm. in diameter) and showing heat symptoms are considered or diagnosed as mid-cycle oestrus.

DO YOU KNOW ?

Temporary Engorgement of Teat (TET) :

TET has relationship with occurrence of oestrus in buffaloes. It is a peculiar phenomenon exhibited by majority of the buffaloes prior to the onset of real heat. The proestrus behaviour is used by most animal owners as an important tool for detection of incoming oestrous. Duration of TET phenomenon is of 3 days.

7. By fern pattern of cervical mucus :

Principle : Sodium and potassium ions / colloids in the mucus when dried, take the shape of fern leaf at high oestrogen levels.

Procedure :

- Take a 18" long glass tube attached to a syringe or use AI gun and disposal sheath.

33

- Pass it in the cervix and aspirate the mucus and collect in a test tube (or cut a piece of hanging cervical mucus from the vulva with a pair of scissors.)
- Take a drop of cervical mucus on a glass slide and spread it evenly.
- Dry it in air or gently warm over the flame.
- Examine the slide under low power (10 X) microscope and note the crystallization pattern.
- Characteristic fern-like patterns (crystallization pattern) are visible under the microscope. Different fern patterns are exhibited at different stages of oestrus.
- These patterns are absent in the mucus drawn during luteal phase and from pregnant animals.

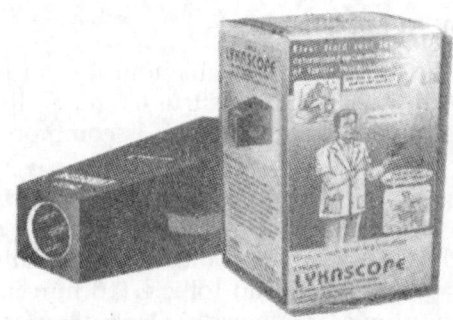

Fig. 4.2 : Lykascope

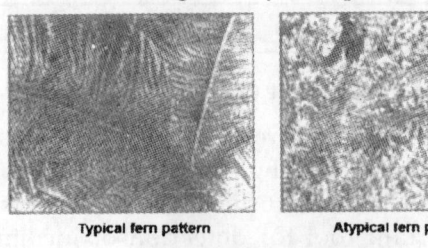

Typical fern pattern   Atypical fern pattern

Nil type

Fig. 4.3 : Showing different types of fern patterns.

- However, pregnant animals which exhibit symptoms of oestrus, show crystallization pattern in cervical mucus.
- The fern pattern can be classified into three types (see Fig. 4.3).
  - **Typical** – Clear fern leaf-like appearance. The branches are well marked and have bright and thick boundaries.
  - **Atypical** – Mixed type appearance. Fern branches remain discontinous and are not well cut out into further branching.
  - **Nil type** – No fern like appearance.

Interpretation :

- **Early heat :** Fern patterns are scattered and are small in size. Branching is thin and fine.
- **Mid heat :** Arborization or crystallization is visible through out the smear. The branches are well marked and have bright and thick boundaries. Tertiary to quaternary or quinquinial branching is observed. This type of pattern is generally referred as "typical".
- **Late heat :** Crystallization is not typical. Fern branches are discontinuous and not well cut out into further branchings. There is an **increased infiltration of lymphocytes in the smear also.**

IMPORTANT POINTS
• In some animals cervical secretion shows fern like pattern even from few days before the actual oestrus to some days after its end. Animals with weaker oestrogenic activity may have thin, scattered and irregular types of crystallization pattern in their cervical mucus.
• There is no vulvar wrinkle in buffaloes as in cow.
• During oestrus in buffaloes, discharge is thin and not copious as in cow.
• Pregnant animals can expel mucus discharge, but it will be more thick, may be moderately cloudy and its tip will be like a 'club'.

Crystoscope : (see Fig. 4.2).

- It is the first field tool for determining optimum time of insemination.
- It is developed by Scientist of I.V.R.I.
- It is available in the market with diferent names (Lykascope etc.).

- It is based on fern pattern of cervical mucus.

Procedure :

- Put the dried slide in the slide gasket of the Lykascope.
- Shift the red button to switch on the light system.
- See the slide through eyepiece.
- Match the fern pattern from the lykascope calender.

CLINICAL CORRELATIONS	
• Interval between two heats is 7-8 days	– Acute endometritis
• Interval between two heats is 10-11 days	– Mid cycle heat
• Interval between two heats is 13-17 days	– Endometritis
• Interval between two heats is 23 to 37 – 45 days	– Embryonic death
• Interval between two heats is 42-45 days	– Missed heat or silent heat
• Interval between two heats is 2-3 days	– Split heat
• Interval between two heats is 4 to 8 days and remained in heat for 2-3 days continuously	– Follicular cyst

DO YOU KNOW ?
In non-pregnant large domestic animals, inflammation of the endometrium due to bacterial infection can result in significant synthesis and release of $PGF_2\alpha$ leading to premature luteolysis and shortening of the oestrous cycle. Thus short oestrous cycle in large domestic animals are pathognomonic sign for uterine infection.

OBSERVATIONS :

Date ....

- Case No. ....
- Age of animal ....
- Signs of heat ...., ..., ..., ...
- Loin reflex (present/absent) ....
- Clitoris massage reflex (present/absent) ....

- Tail reflex   *present/absent*
- Nature of vaginal discharge ....
- Length of vaginal discharge ....
- Fern pattern ....
- Colour of vaginal mucus membrane ....
- Finding of per-rectal examination.
  Cervix ....
  Uterus ....
  Ovary ....
- Diagnosis ....

EXERCISE :

1. What do you understand by 'loin reflex', 'tail reflex' and 'clitoris massage reflex' ?

Ans.

2. How can a trained dog detect heat in cows ?

Ans.

3. How will you diagnose 'mid-cycle heat' by per-rectal examination ?

Ans.

4. What do you understand by TET ?

Ans.

5. Why cervical mucus of oestrus cow get crystallized ?

Ans.

6. What are the differences between 'typical' and 'atypical' fern pattern ?

Ans.

7. What are the different methods of preparation of teaser bull ?

Ans.

❇ ❇ ❇ ❇ ❇

Technology generation is not useful unless it is user-friendly.

Chapter 5

Behavioural Signs of Oestrus in Mare, Ewe, Doe and Bitch

Mare :
- Vicious temperament
- Frequent micturition
- Brownish yellow discharge from vagina
- The tail head is often raised and the clitoris is exposed by frequent **"winking" of the vulva** (sometime called **"winking of clitoris"**)
- The vulvar mucus membrane is congested and become orange or scarlet in colour
- During oestrus, the mare turns her back to the stallion and stands quietly with tail raised to one side

Ewe and Doe :
- Restlessness
- Anorexia
- Homosexual behaviour is exhibited occasionally in goat but not in sheep
- **Frequent and peculiar type of bleating** which is a good sign of heat in doe
- Drop in milk yield
- Swelling of vulva
- **Shaking of tail continuously is also a good sign of heat in doe**
- Oestrus doe prevents other doe to approach or attract the male.
- Signs of oestrus are more clear in does than ewes
- Ewes display a strong ram-seeking behavioural pattern

DO YOU KNOW ?

- Ewes that are not in oestrus usually urinate when a ram approaches whereas oestrus ewes do not. The urination by ewe is a non-contact communication that gives a clue to rams about the oestrus status of the ewe under field conditions. The ewes avoid disturbance by signaling (urination) that they are not sexually receptive.

- Rapid side-to-side or up-and-down tail flagging is a good sign of heat in doe that can be detected in the absence of a buck. This behaviour probably serves to **spread odours** from her vulva to nearby males.

CLINICAL POINTERS

- A common method of heat detection for a small herd of doe is **to rub a rag (small piece of cloth) on the buck's scent glands and store it in a tightly closed container or jar. The jar is opened and presented to the doe each day. If the doe is in oestrus, she will show great interest in the jar.**

- As heat progresses in a doe, a variable amount of transparent mucus is visible in the cervix and on the floor of the vagina (can be seen by speculum examination). This mucus later turns cloudy and finally cheesy white at the end of heat.

- Conception is best when a doe is bred at the stage in which her cervical mucus is cloudy.

SOW :
- Restlessness
- Mounting on other animals
- Lordosis
- Vulvar swelling
- Pink red colour vulva
- Mucus discharge occasionally
- Low-pitched growl
- Onset of frequent tail wagging is the most useful trait for detecting the onset of oestrus

To ensure adequate expression of heat in gilts and sows that are to be mated, they should be housed near (but not too close) to the mature boars. Housing opposite to boars with a 1.0 metre or more wide corridor between the two pens appears suitable.

BACK-PRESSURE TEST

- Back-pressure test or riding test or lordosis is most efficient and practical method of oestrus detection in the sow.
- The efficiency of this test is greatly enhanced if the females are adjacent to boars (at the place where they receive intense boars stimulation).
- Separation from boars by as little as 1 metre can reduce the efficiency of the test.
- **Intense olfactory, auditory and visual stimuli** from the boar facilitate the standing response of oestrus females to pressure on their back.
- The oestrus females which are kept very close to boars by a wire-mesh only receive continuous and intense stimulation from the boars, those females reduce the standing response to the "back-pressure test".
- Therefore, males should be kept opposite to the females pen at a distance of 1 meter wide corridor. But during the back-pressure test, the male should be kept adjacent to the females where they receive boar stimulation (i.e only separated by a wiremesh wall).
- The attendant should quietly approach and apply hand pressure or sitting pressure gently but firmly on the mid region of back of the female.
- **It is useful to massage the flanks** of the females manually prior to applying pressure to the back.

Bitch :

- The vulvar discharge becomes less haemorrhagic, even colourless than pro-oestrus period.
- The vulvo-vaginal swelling is maximum and soft.
- During the pro-oestrus period, the bitch remains attractive to the dog but she does not stand for him and generally attacks him if he attempts to mount her.
- During oestrus period, her attitude changes and she shows signs of courtship towards the male.
- When a male attempts to mount, most oestrus bitches will deviate the tail from the midline and stand to be bred.
- **Tail turning reflex :** When the **perineum** of the oestrus bitch is massaged, even the bitches of poor libido usually respond with tail movement and keen bitches may adopt an exaggerated standing posture with very marked deflection of the tail.

EXERCISE :

1. What are the characteristic symptoms of heat in doe ?

Ans.

2. What are the typical symptoms of heat in mare ?

Ans.

3. What is the typical symptom of heat in sow.

Ans.

4. What indicates an ewe by urinating when a ram approaches to her ?

Ans.

5. Where is buck's scent gland situated ?

Ans.

6. How will you detect heat in a herd of doe without using teaser ?

Ans.

7. What is the colour of vaginal discharge of bitch during proestrous period ?

Ans.

8. What is the colour of vaginal discharge of a bitch during heat ?

Ans.

9. Why does a doe keep flagging her tail during oestrus?

Ans.

10. In which stage, a doe should be bred for better conception rate?

Ans.

11. What should be the location of boar's and sow's pen ?

Ans.

12. Why does an oestrus sow show standing response to back pressure?

Ans.

❊ ❊ ❊ ❊ ❊

Efficiency is the capacity to bring proficiency into expression.

- Swami Chinmayananda

Chapter 6

Detection of Oestrus in Bitch by Vaginal Cytology

OBJECTIVE :

To manage a successful breeding between a bitch and a stud dog.

PRINCIPLE :

The principle of vaginal cytology is simple. The vaginal epithelium is sensitive to levels of oestradiol and it changes from a **bistratified cuboidal epithelium** to a **stratified squamous epithelium** of greater than 30 cell layers. Thereafter these cells slowly mature, keratinized and fall in vaginal lumen (exfoliate).

MATERIALS REQUIRED :

Slides, blunted glass pipette with rubber bulb or sterile cotton-swabs, isotonic saline solution, stain (Leishman's or methylene blue or Giemsa), microscope etc.

PROCEDURE :

(A) Sample collection :
- **Pipette method :**
  - Take 1ml isotonic solution into the pipette.
  - The pipette is inserted into vagina.
  - Squeeze bulb of the pipette several times to mix the vaginal discharge with isotonic solution.
  - Suck the vaginal discharge and withdraw the pipette.
  - Take a small drop of fluid from the pipette on the slide.
  - Tip the slide vertically to allow the drop to run down the length of the slide.
  - Blot the excess fluid from the end of slide and air dry.
- **Swab method :**
  - A cotton swab is moistened with saline solution.

- Insert the speculum into the vagina.
- Insert the cotton swab in the vagina and twist a full turn to pick up a sample of cells.
- Withdraw the swab.
- Place the swab on the slide and roll it over the surface of slide.
- Dry in air.

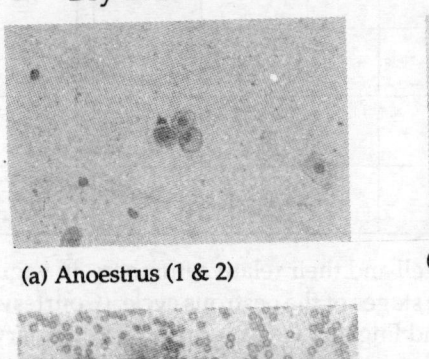

(a) Anoestrus (1 & 2)

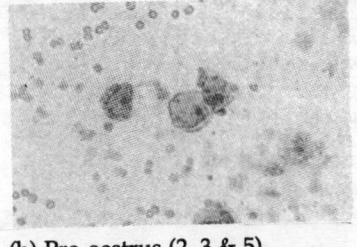

(b) Pro-oestrus (2, 3 & 5)

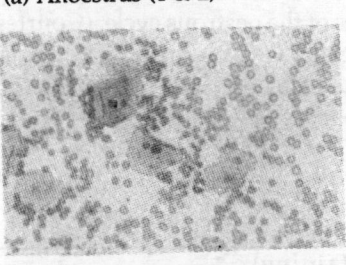

(c) Eary oestrus (3, 4 & 5)

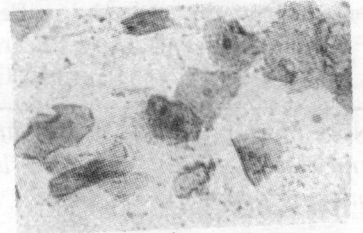

(d) Oestrus (3, 4 & 5). Percentage of anuclear cells is high

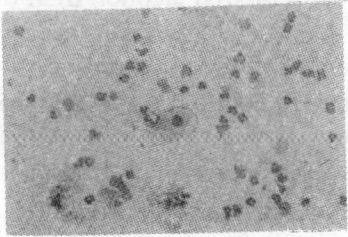

(e) Metoestrus (2 & 6)

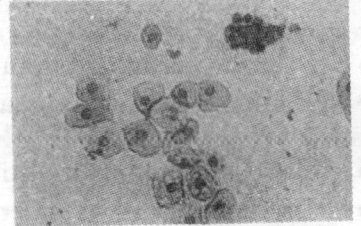

(f) Late metoestrus (1 & 2)

Fig. 6.1: Photomicrographs of exfoliative vaginal cells during various stages of the reproductive cycle. The smears have been stained with a modified Wright-Giemsa stain. (Courtesy of Noakes, D.E. Parkinson, J.T. and England G.C.W. Arthur's Veterinary Reproduction and Obstetrics).

1. Para basal
2. Small intermediate
3. Large intermediate
4. Anuclear keratinised.
5. RBC
6. Neutrophilis

Cell type		Pro-oestrus Early	Pro-oestrus Late	Oestrus Early	Oestrus Late	Early metoestrus	Anoestrus	Vaginitis pyometra
Para basal		+ + +	+	–	–	–	+ +	±
Small intermediate		+ + +	+ +	–	–	+	+	±
Large intermediate		±	+ +	+ + +	+ + +	–	–	±
Anuclear keratinised		–	+ +	+ + + +	+ + +	±	–	–
Red blood		+	+ + +	+ +	–	–	±	±
Neutrophilis		+	–	–	+	+ + +	+	+ + + +

Fig.6.2 : Changes in the types of cell and their relative numbers, in vaginal smears from the bitch during the stages of the oestrous cycle. (Courtesy of Noakes, D.E. Parkinson, J.T. and England G.C.W. Arthur's Veterinary Reproduction and Obstetrics).

Note : *Swab method is somewhat more uncomfortable for the bitch and also deeper cells come in the sample. This causes confusion during interpretation.*

(B) Slide Staining : (Leishman's staining)

- Fix the smear for several seconds in methyl alcohol, then dry in air before staining.
- Pour the Leishman's solution on the slide for 1 minute.
- Dilute the stain with equal volume of distilled water and leave it for 10-15 minutes.
- Wash the slide with distilled water.
- Dry it and observe under oil immersion lens (100X).

Interpretation :

Different types of cells are found in vaginal smear due to desquamation of epithelial cells during pro-oestrus and oestrus (see Fig. 6.1 & 6.2 photographs). These are-

(i) **Parabasal cell** : It is round cells with relatively **large nucleus**.

(ii) **Small intermediate cell** : It is larger than parabasal cells but have **relatively small nucleus**.

(iii) **Large intermediate cell** : It is larger and **irregular** than small intermediate cell but have relatively **small nucleus**.

44

(iv) Anuclear keratinised cell : It is **irregular in shape** and have either **very small or no nucleus.**

Thus, we see that as the epithelial cells mature, their nucleus to cytoplasmic ratio gradually decline.

(v) RBC.

(vi) Neutrophils.

Interesting Fact

Female Old World monkey have a "sex skin" (perianal skin). Under the influence of oestrogen the "Sex skin" becomes hyperaemic and swells. Oestrogen levels increase at the time of oestrus making their posterior bright red. This serves as a visual signal to male, "announcing" the optimum time for copulation.

OBSERVATIONS :   Date : ....

- Case No. ....
- Age ....
- Breed ....
- Nature of vaginal discharge   *serosanguineous/clear*
- Condition of vulva   *swollen/turgid/both*
- Reaction to male   *attract/receptive/non-receptive*
- Finding of vaginal smear.............., ..., ...

EXERCISE :

1. Desquamation of epithelial cells occurs during pro-oestrus and oestrus period. Give reason.

Ans.

2. Mature epithelial cells die and get converted into anuclear keratinized cells. Give reason.

Ans.

3. Neutrophils remain absent during late pro-oestrus and early oestrus. Give reason.

Ans.

4. RBCs are seen in large numbers during early pro-oestrus and decrease over time throughout pro-oestrus and oestrus. Give reason.

Ans.

5. In which stage of oestrous cycle of bitch, maximum numbers of keratinized cells are found ?

Ans.

6. Collection of vaginal discharge by pipette method is better than swab method. Why ?

Ans.

7. Neutrophils again appear in late oestrus and early metoestrus. Give reason.

Ans.

8. Which one is the least mature epithelial cell in vaginal smear?

Ans.

9. Which one is the fully mature epithelial cell in vaginal smear ?

Ans.

❈ ❈ ❈ ❈ ❈

Some books are to be tasted, others to be swallowed and some to be chewed and digested.
— *Bacon.*

Chapter 7

Gynaecological Examination of Vagina

OBJECTIVE :

To know the physiological and pathological condition of vagina.

MATERIALS REQUIRED : Vaginal speculum, liquid paraffin, soap, water etc.

PROCEDURE :

- Restrain the cow in a crate or trevis.
- Clean the vulva and adjacent parts with cotton dipped in normal saline or antiseptic solution.
- Lubricate the sterilized vaginal speculum with liquid paraffin or soap water.
- Insert the speculum through the vulva into vagina while keeping the jaws of speculum closed to avoid injury.
- Turn the handle of vaginal speculum either downward or upward and open the jaws.
- Use torch to observe the anterior part of vagina and outer part of cervix.
- Note the finding like discharge, vaginitis, abscess, tumour, cervix (open or closed), cervicitis etc.
- Remove the speculum in an open fashion.

INTERESTING FACTS

- Speculum examination is totally contra-indicated in pregnant animals and in animals suffering from severe vaginitis and other painful conditions.
- Vaginal examination, AI or intrauterine treatment is contraindicated when the vulvar lips are wet or soiled.

OBSERVATIONS :

Date : ....

- Case No. ....
- Species ....
- History ....
- Condition of vagina — *Normal/Swollen*
- Colour of mucus membrane — ....
- Nature of discharge — ....
- Abnormal condition, if any — ....
- Cervix — *Closed/Open*
- Diagnosis ....
- **Treatment**

Rx

1.
2.
3.
4.

EXERCISE :

1. How will you confirm that animal is in oestrus during examination of vulva ?

Ans.

2. Removal of vaginal speculum should be in an open fashion. Give reason.

Ans.

3. Vaginal speculum is inserted in a closed fashion. Give reason.

Ans.

4. How painting of cervix of an anoestrus cow is performed ?

Ans.

5. Write the composition of Lugol's iodine.

Ans.

It does not take much strength to do things, but it requires great strength to decide on what to do. - ***Elbert Hubbard.***

Chapter 8

Technique of Intra-uterine Therapy

OBJECTIVE :

To introduce the drugs into the uterus to overcome the infection in various disease conditions.

MATERIALS REQUIRED :

Obel's apparatus, catheter, syringe, cotton, saline, pipettes, etc.

PROCEDURE :

- Clean vulva and perineal region with the dry cotton.
- Insert the left hand in the rectum and remove the faecal material by back racking.
- Spread vulva apart and insert the instrument (catheter or Obel's apparatus) up to fornix.
- Hold the cervix between two fingers through rectal wall and keep thumb on the external os.
- The catheter is initially inserted pointing upwards at an angle of about 30^0 to avoid entering into the external urethral opening and is then moved horizontally until it is engaged in the external os of the cervix.
- Entry into the external os is accompanied by a characteristic 'gritty' sensation.
- Thereafter, introduce the catheter through convoluted cervical canal by manipulation of the cervix through rectal wall.
- Place one finger over the internal os of the cervix, so that the tip of the catheter can be palpated when it passes the cervical canal.
- As soon as, the catheter is passed, the drug should be pushed through syringe into the body of uterus not in uterine horn.
- In this way, drug is equally distributed between the two uterine horns.

IMPORTANT POINTS

- The recto-vaginal method of intrauterine medication requires considerable practice for success.
- Obstruction in passing catheter by vaginal folds can be minimized by pushing the cervix forward. By doing this, vaginal passage becomes unfolded.
- After passing catheter in the cervix, no forward pressure should be exerted on the catheter with the right hand because uterine wall is friable and easily penetrated if the catheter moves suddenly.
- **The most common fault during intra uterine therapy is twisting of cervix in the left hand which occuludes uterine horns.**

INTERESTING FACTS

- The irritant solutions or antibiotics, such as Lugol's iodine, tetracycline, etc., when given intrauterine, affects the length of oestrous cycle.
- The irritant intrauterine infusions given during days 3 to 9 of the cycle (oestrus day 0) may significantly shorten the time for the female to return in oestrus.
- The infusions at oestrus or mid-diestrus does not affect oestrous cycle length.
- The infusions on days 14 to 17 of the cycle (oestrus day 0) prolong the luteal period or oestrous cycle length.

OBSERVATIONS :

Date : ....

- Case No. ....
- Species ....
- Age of animal ....
- History of animal ....
- Problems of animal ....
- Drug chosen for IU ....

EXERCISE :

1. Write the commonly used intrauterine drugs, their indications and doses?

Ans.

2. Intrauterine therapy is contraindicated in case of acute puerperal metritis. Give reason.

Ans.

3. Why the DIS (dilute iodine solution) does not affect the oestrous cycle length when given intrauterine during oestrus and mid-diestrus?

Ans.

4. How does the DIS shorten the length of oestrous cycle when given intrauterine during days 3 to 9 of the cycle ?

Ans.

5. How does the DIS lengthen the length of oestrous cycle when it is given intrauterine during days 14 to 17 of the cycle ?

Ans.

❈ ❈ ❈ ❈ ❈

Books are the treasured wealth of the world, the fit inheritance of generations and nations. — **Bacon.**

Chapter 9

Collection of Genital Discharge

OBJECTIVE :

To examine the genital discharge to have an idea about different types of infections, severity of condition, diagnosis and its treatment.

MATERIALS REQUIRED :

Catheter, pipette, cotton gauze, syringe and sterilized bottle.

METHODS :

A. **By back racking -**
    - After inserting the hand into rectum, slightly lift the uterus and cervix upward and massage in backward direction.
    - Thereafter, massage backwardly to the vagina through rectal wall which will result in flow of cervical mucus through the vulvar lips.
    - Collect the discharge in a wide-mouthed sterilized test tube.
    - Cut the discharge with the help of scissors when it remains hanging.

B. **By catheter/pipette :**
    - Introduce the catheter into vagina (anterior part) or cervix or from where genital discharge has to be collected.
    - Suck the mucus with the help of syringe which remains attached to the other end of catheter or pipette.

C. **Tampon method :**
    - Take a sterile gauze tampon of about 1 g. and attach a string to it.
    - Insert the sterilized gauze tampon into the vagina.
    - Leave the tampon in the vagina for 20 min.

- Remove the tampon from the vagina by pulling the string.
- Place it in a sterilized bottle containing saline.

EXERCISE :

1. Which stage of oestrous cycle is the most appropriate time for collection of genital discharge ?

Ans.

2. Enlist the different methods of collection of vaginal discharge ?

Ans.

The true meaning of life is to plant trees whose shade you do not expect to sit.

Chapter 10

Examination of Cervico-Vaginal Mucus Sample

Examination of cervico-vaginal mucus sample help in the assessment of physio-pathological condition of female genital organs.

1. **Colour**
    - Transparent – Normal (in oestrus period).
    - Scanty reddish colour discharge – Metoestrus phase
    - Opaque or transparent with flakes – Mild infection
    - White or yellow colour – Metritis/ pyometra

2. **Consistency**
    - Thin watery – Early oestrus
    - Viscous and ropy – Mid heat
    - Thick – Late heat

3. **Odour** – Normally, genital discharge is odourless. However, foul smelling odour generally indicates severe metritis with systemic involvement with possible retention of foetal membrane or some foetal parts in the uterus. It is usually found in case of post- parturient disorder.

4. **pH** : The pH of genital discharge can be recorded by an ordinary pH indicator paper or using pH meter. The normal pH of genital discharge ranges from **6.5 to 7.4**. A higher pH indicates presence of infection.

5. **White side test** :
    - Take 1 ml. cervical mucus in a sterilized test tube.
    - Add 1 ml 5% sodium hydroxide solution to it.
    - Heat the mixture upto its boiling point.

Interpretation :
    - Dark yellow colour – Clinical metritis

- Yellow colour – Subclinical metritis
- No colour – Normal
6. **Microbiological examination :** The discharge is sent for isolation and identification of organisms and for antibiotic sensitivity test.

OBSERVATIONS :

Date : ....

- Case No. ....
- Species ....
- Breed ....

Physical examination :

- Colour ....
- Consistency ....
- Nature (serous/mucus/muco-purulent) ....
- Presence of blood   Yes/No
- Odour ....
- pH ....

Microscopic examination

- Fern pattern   *Present/Absent*   *Typical/Atypical*
- RBC   *Present/Absent*
- Protozoa   *Present/Absent*   if present, species ....

White side test (Colour) ....

Bacteriological examination.

Micro organism (s) ....

Most sensitive drug ....

Diagnosis ....

Treatment

Rx

1.   ....
2.   ....
3.   ....

EXERCISE :

1. What is the importance of White side test ?

Ans.

2. pH of vaginal discharge increases during infection. Give reason.

Ans.

3. What is metoestrus bleeding ?

Ans.

4. What is pro-oestrus bleeding ?

Ans.

Purity, patience and perseverance are the three essentials to success in life and above all Love and Service.

Chapter 11

External and Per-rectal Pregnancy Diagnosis in Bovine

OBJECTIVES :

● The main purpose of pregnancy diagnosis is to detect the non-pregnant ones so that time lost as the result of infertility is reduced significantly either by early breeding or treatment.

● To differentiate the pregnancy and abnormal conditions of the uterus.

MATERIALS REQUIRED :

Full hand sleeve, lubricant, soap, antiseptic solution, gumboots, animal crate, etc.

A.   EXTERNAL EXAMINATION :

(a)   Visual examination :

● Cessation of oestrous cycle after artificial/ natural insemination.

● Sluggish and docile behaviour.

● **Fattening tendency** particularly during early pregnancy.

● Gradual drop in milk yield (after 5 months)

● Gradual increase in body weight.

● Gradual increase in the size of the abdomen.

● **Flanks become hollow and spine appears more prominent.**

● **The size of mammary glands/ udder begins to increase from about 5th months of gestation in heifers, while in older cows it is usually observed just 2-3 weeks before parturition.**

● In few animals, a prepartum **udder oedema** and **umbilical oedema** is noticed.

(b) Abdominal ballotment :

- Abdominal ballotment of foetus on the right side of the animal can be done from 7th **month onwards** (Fig. 11.1).

- Press abdomen (Rt. side) by closed fist and release suddenly and apply the palm against the abdominal wall to feel the foetus which hits the palm.

- A 7th month foetus is felt very near to the ribs and 9th month foetus is felt near the udder.

- Therefore, abdominal ballotment should be performed at proper site as mentioned above.

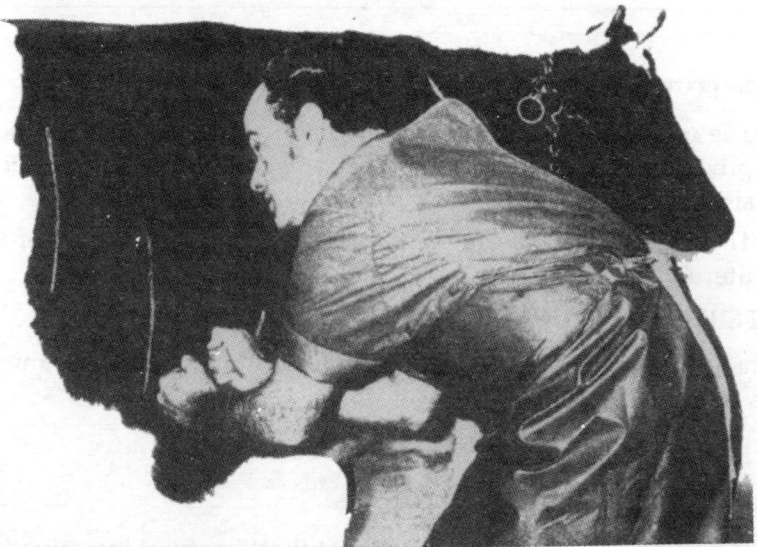

Fig. 11.1 : Rough estimation of the month of pregnancy by means of deep palpation of the flank, using clenched fists. (Courtesy of Rosenberger, G. 1977. Clinical Examination of Cattle. Berlin and Hamburg.)

(c) Drenching cold water :

- Drenching cold water causes the foetal movement **from 7th month onwards.**

- In the early morning, the animal is faced towards north and cold water is drenched or the animal is allowed to drink cold water.

- Examiner should stand near the head of the animal.

- When sun-rays fall on the abdomen, the foetal movement can be well-appreciated in pregnant animal.

(B) PER – RECTAL EXAMINATION (see Fig. 11.2, 11.3, 11.4, 11.5 & 11.6) :

First month (Negative stage) –
- Both the uterine horns are symmetrical.
- Uterine horns are intrapelvic.
- Feel of uterine horn is normal.
- One of the ovaries exhibits CL.
- Cervix remains closed.

Second month (31st to 60th days) or small sac stage :
- Uterus is usually intra-pelvic and palpable from all the sides.
- Uterus is tonic.

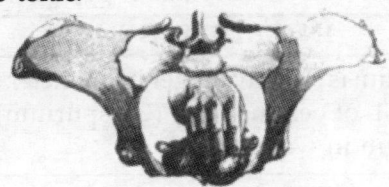

Fig. 11. 2 : Rectal examination of the female genital system in the 70th day of pregnancy. (Courtesy of Benesch, F. and Wright, J.G. 2001. Veterinary Obstetries. Greenworld Publishers).

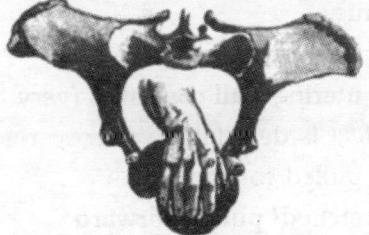

Fig. 11. 3 : Rectal examination of the female genital system in the 90th day of pregnancy. (Courtesy of Benesch, F. and Wright, J.G. 2001. Veterinary Obstetries. Greenworld Publishers).

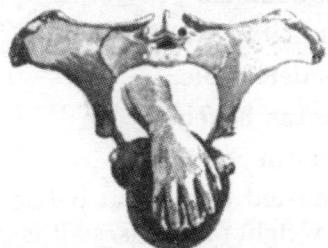

Fig. 11. 4 : Rectal examination of the female genital system in the 110th day of pregnancy. (Courtesy of Benesch, F. and Wright, J.G. 2001. Veterinary Obstetries. Greenworld Publishers).

- Pregnant horn is 2-4 times enlarged.
- **Slippery feel of foetal membrane** when horn is palpated between fingers (double wall) from the 5th **week of pregnancy in heifers** and from the 6th **week in cows (placental palpation).**
- Uterine wall thinner than normal due to increased diameter of uterine horn.
- Ovaries are at normal position and one of the ovary exhibits pregnancy CL or corpus luteum verum, which differs from periodic corpus luteum in not having a neck.
- Cervix is closed and normal in position.

INTERESTING FACT
Corpus luteum verum is slightly longer in diameter (2.5 cm) and weight (6.5 gm) than the CL of oestrus cycle (CL spurium) which is 2.3 cm in diameter and 5.7 gm in weight.

Third month (61st – 90th days) or large sac stage :

- Now, uterus hangs on the brim of pelvis and is palpable from only three sides.
- Uterus is tonic
- Pregnant horn is further enlarged.
- Thinning of uterine wall continues (very thin).
- Rebound effect is detectable.
- Ovaries are pulled forward.
- **Cervix is stretched/ pulled forward.**
- Heaviness is felt when cervix is bulled by examiner.

Fourth month (91st – 120th days) or Balloon stage –

- **Uterus is abdominal.**
- Thinning of uterine wall continues.
- **Cotyledons detectable.**
- Fluctuations can be felt.
- **Fremitus (+) can be felt.**
- Cervix is located beyond/ at pelvic brim (reason-due to increase in weight of uterus, so it is pulled forward).
- **Ovaries are pulled forward and are out of reach i.e. in abdominal cavity.**

Fifth month (121st – 150th days) or sinking stage.
- Uterus is sinking in abdomen.
- Foetus and fluctuations are felt.
- Cotyledons are bigger in size (3.5cm)

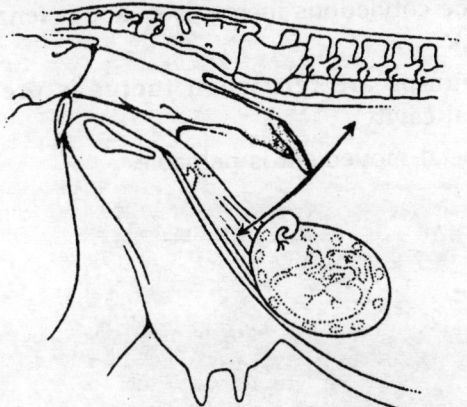

Fig. 11.5 : Rectal examination of the female genital system in the last of 5th month of pregnancy. Neither placentomes, placental membranes nor foetus can be palpated.

- Fremitus (++) can easily be felt.

Sixth to seventh month (151st –210th days) :
- Uterus is entirely abdominal.
- Foetus sinks more deep in the abdominal cavity and is not palpable.
- But in the last of seventh month, foetus starts to come near the pelvic cavity and is easily palpable.
- Fremitus (+++) is strong.

IMPORTANT POINTS

- Pregnancy diagnosis is easy in heifers than cows.
- Early pregnancy diagnosis (35th – 45th days) by inexperienced clinician may results into abortion.

Reason : Excess pressure applied during manipulation of the amniotic vesicles and embryo results rupture of amniotic vesicles and embryonic death. The most common cause of embryonic death is rupture of the heart or the vessels at the base of the heart resulting in haemorrhage into amniotic cavity.

Eight to ninth month (211st – 270th days) :

- Foetus comes again nearer to the pelvic cavity.
- **Foetal parts can be clearly felt.**
- Fremitus (++++) is very strong.
- Size of the cotyledons increases to about **tennis ball size (7 – 8cm.).**
- **Foetal bumps are felt when foetus** is pressed in the abdominal cavity.
- Strong foetal movement is palpable.

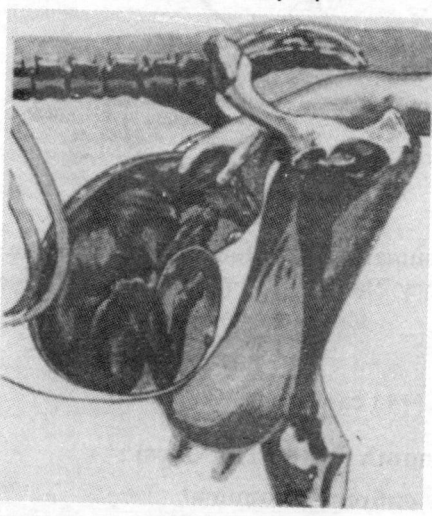

Fig. 11.6 : Rectal examination of the female genital system when pregnancy approaching term. (Courtesy of Benesch, F. and Wright, J.G. 2001. Veterinary Obstetries. Greenworld Publishers).

Slipping of foetal membrane :

- Early pregnancy diagnosis (**from 35 to 90 days**) can be best performed by **palpating foetal membrane.** However **slipping of foetal membrane** occurs through out gestation from 35 days but in late stage of gestation other things are more important than slipping of foetal membranes.
- The technique consists of gently picking up and pinching or compressing pregnant horns of the uterus and feeling the foetal membranes (**chorio-allantois**) which slip between the thumb and the fingers before the uterine wall escaped from between the fingers.
- This technique of slipping the membranes is especially valuable

in the differential diagnosis of pregnancy from uterine disease such as pyometra and mucometra.

- It is important to note that the entire diameter of each uterine horn must be palpated so that if foetal membrane slip is present, it will not be missed.

Palpation of amniotic vesicle :

- From approximately **30 to 65 days of gestation,** the amniotic vesicle can be detected as a movable oval object within the uterine lumen.

- The vesicle is turgid in early pregnancy but becomes **flaccid** with advancing gestation (after 65 to 70 days) when it is difficult to detect at all.

Palpation of placentomes :

- The presence of placentomes is another positive sign of pregnancy.

- These are detectable from **about 75 days to term.**

- These are palpated as soft, thickened lumps in the uterine wall and more easily detected as pregnancy advances.

- In general, the placentomes in the middle of the gravid horn and nearest the attachment of the middle uterine artery are **larger** than those placentomes in the cervical or apical end of the horn or in the opposite horn.

Palpation of foetus :

- The foetus can be palpated from the time of **amniotic softening (65 to 70 days) to term.**

- Palpation of foetus **before 60 to 70 days of gestation is not possible** because of the tense and distended amniotic vesicle, and the small size of the foetus.

- After 60 to 70 days in heifer and small breeds of cow, foetus can be palpated throughout gestation period.

- In heavy breeds of cow, foetus may not be palpable in mid-gestation. In that condition, pregnancy diagnosis is based on the position of the uterus, the size of uterine artery, palpation of placentomes and slipping of foetal membrane.

- After the sixth month of pregnancy, **foetal movement can be stimulated by pinching the claws of foetus, grasping and** pulling of foetal leg, pinching the eye balls or grasping the nose of the foetus through rectal wall.

Palpation of fremitus :

- The major blood supply to the gravid uterus is the **middle uterine artery**; which gets enlarged considerably as pregnancy progresses.

- The blood supply to the left horn is by **left middle uterine artery** and the blood supply to the right horn is by **right middle uterine artery.**

Origin :

- The uterine artery is originated from the **pudendal artery** at the level of the iliac shaft and travel in the broad ligaments.

- Because of their location in the broad ligaments, they are **freely movable** and can be differentiated from the external iliac arteries which are tighly attached to the medial shaft of each ilium.

- Thus, one should not confuse with the **external iliac artery** (it also passes through shaft of ilium) because it **does not move when pulled while middle uterine artery moves when pulled.**

Technique of palpation :

- The **right middle uterine artery** can be palpated by **directly applying fingers** over the right lateral wall of the pelvic cavity and its inlet while the **left middle uterine artery** is examined by **rotating the hand in a clockwise direction** and applying finger over the left lateral wall of the pelvic cavity and its inlet.

- In pregnant animal, a sensation is felt like when a **person presses a rubber pipe for partial obstruction of water flow.** This sensation or turbulence created by blood flow is called **fremitus or whiring or thrill.**

- In early pregnancy, it may be necessary to place very slight pressure on the artery to elicit the fremitus, but as pregnancy progresses the **buzzing becomes obvious without pressure.**

Importance :

- Fremitus gives idea about the horn containing foetus.
- Enlargement of ipsilateral middle uterine artery to the pregnant horn is detectable after 90 days of gestation.
- **By approximately 120 days,** the blood flow within the ipsilateral middle uterine artery has increased to the point at which **turbulence is palpable as a buzzing sensation,** also referred to as a thrill or fremitus.
- The middle uterine artery which supplies blood to the non-pregnant horn, also increases in thickness but the change is slower than the artery of pregnant horn.
- By about 7 to 8 months, the fremitus is often palpable in the contralateral uterine artery.
- **The presence of bilateral fremitus before 7 to 8 months,** especially when the two arteries are symmetrical, this feature strongly suggests **bicornual twins.**
- **If the fremitus was felt in earlier pregnancy and then disappears indicates death of the foetus.**

INTERESTING FACT
Due to increase in the diameter of middle uterine artery the arterial wall becomes thinner as pregnancy advances. Blood flow also increases as pregnancy advances. This is why, instead of feeling a pulsation in the artery (normally) a characteristic 'fremitus' is felt.

IMPORTANT POINTS
• The uterus of heifers is usually located in the pelvic cavity until 3 to 4 months of pregnancy. • In all ages of cattle, the uterus lies on the floor of the abdominal cavity after the 4th month of pregnancy. • From 5th to 6th month of pregnancy, the uterus sinks deeply in the abdomen so that in the larger breeds, only cervix and middle uterine artery (fremitus) can be palpated *per rectum.* • From 6th to 7th month, the foetus becomes large enough so that it can be again palpated on rectal examination in almost all cows. • From 8th to 9th month, the foetus may extend caudally so that nose and feet are resting in the pelvic cavity.

OBSERVATIONS :

Date ....

Breeding history : ....

Visual examination :
- Behaviour ....
- Fattening tendency ....
- Body weight ....
- Changes in abdomen ....
- Flank ....
- Changes in udder ....

Per-rectal examination :
- Location of cervix ....
- Location of horns ....
- Symmetry of horns ....
- Foetal membrane slip ....
- Foetal fluid ....
- Placentomes ....
- Part of foetus ....
- Foetal movement ....

RESULTS :
- Pregnant/Non pregnant
- Duration of pregnancy ....
- Pregnant horn ....
- Any other remarks ....

EXERCISE :

1. What is a placentome ?
Ans.

2. From which months of pregnancy, the slipping of foetal membranes can be noticed ?
Ans.

3. What is a fremitus ?
Ans.

4.   What is the most common cause of embryonic death during early pregnancy diagnosis by an inexperienced clinician ?

Ans.

5.   Cervix becomes flat or stretched during gestation. Give reason.

Ans.

6.   Why does the uterine wall become thinner as pregnancy advances?

Ans.

7.   In which months of pregnancy the uterus is out of reach ?

Ans.

8.   In which months of pregnancy the placentomes increase up to the size of a tennis ball ?

Ans.

9.   What is the time interval of gestation during which only amniotic vesicle can be palpated ?

Ans.

10. From when palpation of placentomes are possible ?

Ans.

11. From when palpation of foetus is possible ?

Ans.

12. From when slipping of foetal membrane is possible ?

Ans.

13. From which month of pregnancy, fremitus is felt ?

Ans.

14. Why middle uterine artery moves when it is pulled ?

Ans.

15. Why placentomes are larger near the attachment of middle uterine artery ?

Ans.

�֎   ✖   ✖   ✖   ✖

No day is lost which is spent with a worthwhile books.

Chapter 12

Early Pregnancy Diagnosis in Cows by "Milk Ejection Test"

OBJECTIVES :
- To confirm the pregnancy after 20-22 days of insemination.
- To reduce duration of service period.

PRINCIPLE :
$PGF_2\alpha$ in nonluteolytic dose induces the release of oxytocin from the corpus luteum which causes let-down of milk in the lactating and pregnant cows.

PROCEDURE :
- This test is performed generally 3 hrs. prior to the evening milking in dairy cows (18-22 days after insemination).
- Place the teat cannula in the left fore-teat and leave it for milk flow from **teat cistern.**
- When the milk flow ceases, a small dose (2.5 mg or 0.5 ml) of **Dinoprost (Lutalyse)** is administered **intravenously** through ear vein.
- If the corpus luteum of pregnancy is present, **alveolar milk** starts to flow about **one minute later.**

OBSERVATIONS :

Date ....

- Case No.   ....
- Species   ....
- Breed   ....
- Date of service ....
- Time of test   ....
- Dose & route of drug ....
- Finding   ....

EXERCISE :

1. After how many days from oestrus, milk ejection test should be performed and why ?

Ans.

2. What will happen if the milk ejection test is performed before 18 days of insemination ?

Ans.

3. How does $PGF_2\alpha$ help in secretion of oxytocin from the corpus luteum ?

Ans.

4. Why the teat cannula is applied before the administration of non-luteolytic dose of $PGF_2\alpha$?

Ans.

Kindness is a language, which the deaf can hear and the blind can read.
– Mark Twain.

Chapter 13

Differential Diagnosis of Pregnancy in Bovine

OBJECTIVE :

To prevent false positive diagnosis. There are many cases in which uterus remain distended and an in experienced person may make false positive diagnosis.

Pyometra :

- Pus remains present in the uterus.
- Both the uterine horns remain equally distended while in pregnancy, horns remain asymmetrical.
- **Fremitus is absent** in pyometra because there is no need to supply extra blood.
- **Thick uterine wall and lack of tone** while in pregnancy, thin and tonic uterine wall.
- **No dorsal bulging of the horn like as in case of pregnancy because pus tends to gravitate and collect in dependent portions of the horns.**
- Placentomes are absent.
- No slipping of foetal membrane.
- If the diagnosis is uncertain, re-examine after one or two months. In normal pregnancy, progressive development of the foetus and uterus occurs, whereas in pyometra, the condition remains essentially same.

Mucometra or hydrometra :

- No slipping of foetal membrane
- No placentomes
- No fremitus
- Failure of progressive development of uterus as in a normal pregnancy

Mummification :

- Solid mass tightly surrounded by uterine wall.
- No placental fluids.
- **Intra-abdominal uterus may be confused with pregnancy.**
- No increase in the size of abdomen.
- No placentomes
- No fremitus.
- If ovary is palpable, CL is present just like as in pregnancy.

Foetal maceration :

- No fremitus
- No placentomes
- Cervix is partially closed
- Skeletal part of foetus keeps on floating within lumen of uterus which gives a **characteristics crepitating feeling or gritty feeling**

INTERESTING FACTS
• Apart from these conditions, an inexperienced person may confuse with visceral organs of the animal. Ovaries – may be confused with *cotyledons.* Distended ventral sac of rumen - may be confused with *foetus.* Distended urinary bladder – may be confused with *pregnant horns.* • Anatomically, there is no reason for confusing a pregnant uterus with such structures. Careful rectal examination, consideration of the anatomical structures and relationships of these organs and their consistency will prevent erroneous diagnosis.

OBSERVATIONS :

Date ....

- Case No.   ....
- Species   ....
- Breed   ....
- Age   ....
- History   ....
- Per–rectal examination

- Cervix ....
- Uterus ....
- Ovary ....
- Fremitus ....
- Placentomes ....
- Amniotic vesicle ....
- **Diagnosis** ....
- **Treatment**

Rx

1.
2.
3.
4.

EXERCISE :

1. Why dorsal bulging of uterine horn does not occur in pyometra as seen in pregnancy ?

Ans.

2. With which visceral organ, an inexperienced clinician may confuse with foetus?

Ans.

3. With which visceral organ, an inexperienced clinician may confuse with urinary bladder ?

Ans.

4. With which reproductive organ, an inexperienced clinician may confuse with cotyledons ?

Ans.

As land is improved by sowing with various seeds, so is the mind by exercising with different studies.

Chapter 14

Pregnancy Diagnosis in Small Ruminants

I. Recto-abdominal palpation technique : (see Fig. 14.1)

A simple and reliable technique for diagnosing pregnancy and detection of multiple pregnancy in small ruminants (sheep & goat) is of paramount importance for field veterinarians.

Materials Required : Soap enema, lubricator, glass or steel rod (50 cm. long and 1.5 cm. in diameter), test tube, etc.

Principle : This method is based on detecting the enlarged pregnant uterus by means of a probe inserted into the rectum. This procedure is **reliable after mid-pregnancy.**

Procedure :

- A soap enema is given 5 minutes before examination to evacuate the rectum.
- The ewe or doe is restrained on her back.
- A lubricated glass or steel rod (50 cm long and 1.5 cm. in diameter) is carefully inserted approximately 30 cm. inside the rectum.
- Left palm is placed on the abdominal wall and the rod is moved to and fro and side to side in a horizontal plane with the right hand.
- If the distal end of rod is palpable in the region of uterus with no obstruction across the abdomen, the ewe or doe is considered non-pregnant.
- If a palpable mass is detected in place of distal end of rod by the free hand over abdominal wall on one or both sides, the ewe or doe is considered pregnant.
- The number of foetuses are assessed according to the size and position of palpable mass.

Accuracy : Accuracy ranges from **90-100%**. Inaccuracies can result due to involuting uterus where history of abortion or parturition was not known.

II. Abdominal palpation :

Procedure :

- Withhold feed and water for 12-24 hrs. before abdominal palpation.
- The ewe or doe is restrained in a sitting position.
- One hand is placed against the left abdomen.
- Right abdomen is palpated by using finger-tips.
- The foetus is felt as a floating body when it is pushed away and then returned to the finger-tips.

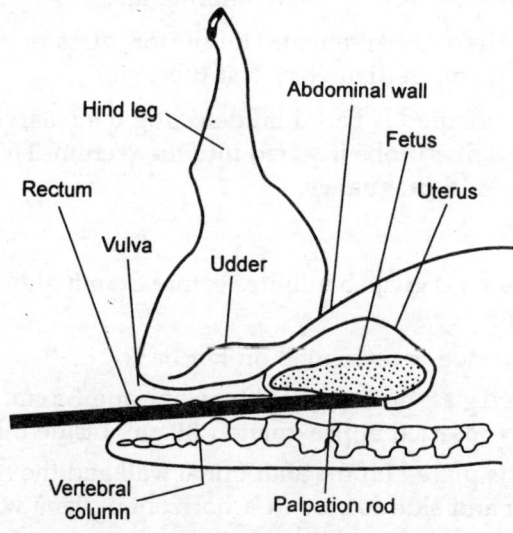

Fig. 14.1 : Longitudinal section illustrating recto-abdominal palpation technique in an ewe. The animal is turned on her back.

Different foetal ballotment techniques are used by field veterinarians. These are :

- By sitting one side of the animal, raise the abdomen just in front of udder with one hand whilst with other hand's fingers, push the abdomen from flank towards the hand used to lift. The foetus is felt as a floating body in pregnant animal.

- Raise the abdomen just in front of udder by taking the hand between hind legs whilst with other hand, push the abdomen from flank towards the hand used to lift. Repeat with the other side by changing the hand for lifting and pushing. The foetus is felt as a floating body in pregnant animal.
- Press the abdomen just in front of the stifle joint with edge of palm and swing the animal from side to side, the balloted foetus or foetuses within uterus can be felt.

III. Mammary secretion test :

- This test is efficient, easy to perform, less time consuming, cheap and applicable in field condition.
- Mammary secretion is taken in a test tube by stripping the teats.
- This secretion is rubbed on palm.
- When it is felt **sticky and honey-like**, the ewe or doe is considered pregnant.
- The honey like mammary secretion gives better results **from 70 days of gestation onwards** for detection of pregnancy in doe or ewe.

IV. Palpation of caudal uterine artery per vaginum :

- A fairly reliable method to diagnose pregnancy after 50 days.
- At pregnancy the caudal uterine arteries on the anterior vaginal wall at **10 'o' clock** and **2 'o' clock position** can be palpated by gloved lubricated index and middle fingers.
- In the non-pregnant, the arteries are very small and cannot be palpated.

OBSERVATIONS :

Date ....

- Case No. ....
- Species ....
- Breed ....
- Date of last heat/service ....
- Finding of recto-abdominal technique.

Pregnant/Non-pregnant ....

Number of foetus ....

Duration of pregnancy ....

- Finding of mammary secretion test : ....
- Palpation of caudal uterine artery ....

EXERCISE :

1. What is the principle of recto-abdominal technique of pregnancy diagnosis in a doe or ewe ?

Ans.

2. What is the accuracy of recto-abdominal technique of pregnancy diagnosis ?

Ans.

3. After how many days of pregnancy, mammary secretion test gives positive results ?

Ans.

4. What should be the length and diameter of probe used in recto-abdominal technique for pregnancy diagnosis ?

Ans.

5. In which position, the ewe or doe is restrained in abdominal palpation technique for pregnancy diagnosis ?

Ans.

6. In which position, the ewe or doe is restrained in recto-abdominal technique for pregnancy diagnosis ?

Ans.

❋ ❋ ❋ ❋ ❋

Knowledge is a treasure, but practice is the key to it.

Chapter **15**

Biological and Chemical Methods of Pregnancy Diagnosis

Biological methods :

1.   Ascheim Zondek (A-Z) Test : This is a biological test utilized for diagnosis of pregnancy in **mare**. This test is based on FSH like activity of PMSG, present in the blood of pregnant mare. This test is more accurate between **days 50-100 post conception.**

Procedure :
- Collect 30-40 ml. mare's blood from the jugular vein.
- Allow it to coagulate for 24 hours and separate the serum.
- Store the serum at 4⁰C.
- Inject 0.25 ml serum subcutaneously twice daily for 2-4 days to **an immature female rat of about 22 days of age.**
- Kill the rat 96 or 120 hours later and inspect the genital organ.

Interpretation :
If mare is pregnant the genitalia of rat will have following changes.
- **Ovaries –** Many haemorrhagic spots or corpora haemaorrhagica appear as dark-red or black spots.
- **Uterus :**
    - Oedematous.
    - 2 to 4 times of normal size.
    - A little amount of fluid remains present in the uterus.

- **Vagina and Vulva :**
    - Swollen.
    - Vaginal swabs show many cornified epithelial cells.

If mare is not pregnant :

No definite change in ovaries and uterus of rat.

2.   **Friedman test or Rabbit test :**

*   It is not commonly performed because of the cost of rabbit. The basic procedures in this test is similar to rat test but the age of rabbit, the dose of the serum injected will vary.
*   2 ml of mare's serum is injected intravenously in the ear vein of immature female rabbit **(19 to 20 weeks old).**
*   Perform laparotomy after **24 hrs. of injection.**
*   Presence of corpora haemorrhagica in the ovaries and oedematous condition of the uterus indicate positive diagnosis.

Chemical methods :

(i) Cuboni Test :

*   This test is used for pregnancy diagnosis in **mare.**
*   This test involves detection of **oestrogen in the urine of mare** and can be performed **after 150 days of conception.**

Principle – The urine is hydrolysed with HCl, and benzene is added for extraction of oestrogen from hydrolysed urine.

Method -

*   Take 15 ml urine in a test tube and add to it 3 ml conc. HCl.
*   Heat the mixture in a water bath at boiling point for 10 minutes.
*   Cool the mixture.
*   Pour the mixture into a separating funnel and add to it 18 ml benzol and shake well.
*   Collect the benzol layer in an other test tube and add to it 10 ml. conc. H_2SO_4.
*   Heat the mixture at 80^0C for 5 minutes and cool.

Interpretation :

*   Green fluorescence   -   pregnant
*   No colour   -   Non-pregnant

(ii) Barium chloride test :

*   This test is used for pregnancy diagnosis in **cattle and buffalo.**

- It gives more than 90% reliable results.

Principle – End-products of progesterone (after metabolisation in liver) present in the urine and this prevents precipitation of barium chloride while oestrogens favour precipitation.

Method :
- Take 5 ml of urine in a test tube.
- Add 5-6 drops of 1% barium chloride solution and mix well.

Interpretation :
- **Clear white precipitation** : Non-pregnant
- **No precipitation** – Pregnant

Advantage : Pregnancy can be diagnosed even at 3 to 4 weeks of gestation.

Limitation :
- When oestrogens in urine are of plant origin, it may give wrong result.
- Presence of persistent corpus luteum and corpus luteum of pregnancy up to some days after parturition give false positive result.

(iii) Sodium hydroxide test :
- This test is used for pregnancy diagnosis in **cattle and buffalo.**
- This test has a reliability of **80-90%.**

Method
- Take 0.25 ml. of cervical mucus in a test tube.
- Add to it 5 ml 10% solution of NaOH.
- Heat it till boiling.

Interpretation :
- Orange   -   Pregnant
- Pale colour -   Non-pregnant

(iv) Specific gravity method :

This test has more than **90% reliability** both in cows and buffaloes.

Principle – Specific gravity of cervical mucus is increased with progesterone while it is decreased with oestrogens.

Method :

- Take few ml. of copper sulphate solution having specific gravity 1.008 in a test tube.
- Add 0.25 ml cervical mucus in the copper sulphate solution.

Interpretation :

- If mucus sinks - Pregnant
- If mucus floats - Non-pregnant

Seed bio- assay method :

- This method is used for pregnancy diagnosis both in cows and buffaloes.

Principle – Germination of wheat/ barley is prevented by four-fold rise in concentration of **abscicic acid** in the pregnant animals. It induces dormancy in seeds.

Method :

- The urine is collected and diluted four times with distilled water.
- Two petri-dishes are taken and filter papers are placed in it.
- About 15-20 wheat seeds are kept in each petri-dish.
- About 10-15 ml. of the above diluted urine sample is added to one petri-dish, while in other petridish only water is added (control).
- Cover the petri-dishes to prevent evaporation and keep **for 5 days**.

Interpretation :

- No germination and turn black or if germinate but shoots are less than 1cm. in length – **Pregnant.**
- 35-60% germination with moderate shoot length (4 cm.) - **Non-pregnant.**
- **Control petri-dish** – 60-80% germination and shoot length about 6 cm.

EXERCISE :

1. In which animal A-Z test is applied for diagnosis of pregnancy and why ?

Ans.

2. Which laboratory animal is utilized in A-Z test ?

Ans.

3. Why immature female is taken for biological test ?

Ans.

4. In which period of pregnancy A-Z test is most accurate?

Ans.

5. In which animal Cuboni test is applied for diagnosis of pregnancy?

Ans.

6. What are the basis of A-Z test and Cuboni test ?

Ans.

7. After how many days of pregnancy, cuboni test give accurate result ?

Ans.

8. What is the principle of barium chloride test for pregnancy diagnosis ?

Ans.

9. What is the principle of specific gravity method for pregnancy diagnosis?

Ans.

10. After how many days of pregnancy, barium chloride test is suitable for pregnancy diagnosis in cows ?

Ans.

✻ ✻ ✻ ✻ ✻

We must look inwards as happiness is within us, like salt in the ocean.

Chapter 16

Care of the Postpartum Dam

OBJECTIVES :
- To evaluate and identify the postpartum complications.
- Initiation of therapy when it is needed to maximize fertility and lactation.

Care of post partum dam :
- Following parturition, the dam should be allowed to lick and nurse her young.
- Excitement, noise or any unusual happening should be eliminated or prevented.
- The soiled hind quarters and perineum including udder should be cleaned and dried.
- Keep the dam warm to prevent from chill.
- Give warm water and gruel to drink just after parturition.
- Give feed to the cow, first only bran mash moistened with luke warm water to provide **laxative effect**. Some green grass may also be given.
- There are always dangers that high producing cow will develop milk fever and mastitis. To avoid milk fever, complete milk should not be drawn for first 2-3 days. To avoid mastitis, regular test should be done.
- The placenta is normally expelled within 2-4 hours. If it is not expelled by 12 hours then give treatment for expulsion of placenta.
- The amount of grain (bran, oats, maize etc.) should be increased gradually during the first three weeks after parturition to prevent ketosis.
- Excess oedema of the udder should be controlled by massage, frequent milking and by use of diuretics (Frusemide).

- Moderate and light exercise daily should be given after parturition.
- In order to prevent milk fever, incomplete milking is generally practiced but Jersey cattle may become allergic to the α-casein of their own milk and urticaria develop around the udder. This could be treated by prompt and complete milking.
- If genital discharge is purulent in nature, the animal should be treated with suitable antimicrobial agent.
- Sometimes, acute puerperal metritis develop causing septicaemia within 24 to 48 hours post-partum. The symptoms may be severe and death may occur. Any illness occurring immediately after parturition should be treated promptly.
- Agalactia after parturition is noticed occasionally in heifers accompanied with a greatly congested, oedematous and painful udder. Oxytocin (20-30 IU) intravenously or intramuscularly causes rapid and complete milk let-down. Sometimes repeated injection at each milking is required.
- Following a dystocia operation, the genital tract should always be examined for the presence of another foetus in the uterus.
- After every dystocia operation, the genital canal including the uterus should be examined for the presence of an invaginated uterine horn, lacerations or ruptures.
- If the animal is unable to rise, further examination should be made to determine whether obturator paralysis, dislocation of the hips, spinal injuries or milk fever is/are present.

INTERESTING FACT

Milk allergy : Jersey cattle may become allergic to the α-*casein* of their own milk. Normally, this protein is synthesized in the udder and if the animals are milked regularly, nothing untoward occurs. If the milking is delayed, the increased intra-mammary pressure force milk protein back into the blood stream. In allergic cattle, this may cause reactions ranging from mild discomfort with urticarial skin lesions to acute systemic anaphylaxis and death. The condition can be treated by prompt milking. Some seriously affected animals may have to go for several lactations without drying off because of the severe reactions that occur on cessation of milking.

OBSERVATIONS :

Date ....

- Case No. ....
- Species ....
- Breed ....
- Age of animal ....
- Temperature ....
- Pulse rate ....
- Gait of animal ....
- Condition of udder ....
- Placenta *expelled/retained*
- Condition of birth canal ....
- General condition of animal ....
- **Treatment given**

Rx

1.
2.
3.
4.

EXERCISE :

1. What is milk allergy ? Write its line of treatment in a Jersey cow.

Ans.

2. Why should the amount of grain be increased gradually during the first three weets of parturition ?

Ans.

3. How milk fever is prevented ?

Ans.

Concentration and will can be developed as well as muscles; they grow by regular training and exercise. **– *The Mother.***

Chapter **17**

Care of New Born

OBJECTIVE : To reduce the calf mortality at the time of birth.

Care of new born :

During intrauterine life, the foetus is nursed entirely by the dam. At birth, the maternal connections are severed due to rupture of umbilical cord resulting in cessation of nutrient and oxygen supply to foetus. Various measures can be taken to reduce new-born mortality.

1. **To initiate respiration :**
   - Remove mucus from the nostril and mouth with the help of fingers.
   - Draw out the tongue to and fro.
   - Blow air into the nostrils.
   - Vigorously rub the chest with a gunny bag or towel. This tactile stimulus may stimulate respiration.
   - Hold the hind legs of newborn and swing backward and forward resulting in discharge of copious quantity of fluid or mucus from the larger bronchii, throat and nose. (See Fig. 17.1)
   - Pinch the foetal nose.
   - **Tickling the nasal mucosa with straw.**
   - If all the above methods fail, respiration can be stimulated by quickly **giving 40-100 mg Doxapram hydrochloride** to the calf by **intravenous injection or sub -lingual injection.**
   - If respiration is not started even after administration of **Doxapram hydrochloride** but cardiac function is present, then artificial respiration should be attempted.
   - The upper chest wall is raised and lowered, holding it by the humerus and the last rib. This may help to achieve the

strong negative intrathoracic pressure required for the first breath.

Note : *Excessive pressure should not be applied externally to the ribs to avoid the possibility of fracture or damage of underlying organs such as lungs and liver.*

- If spontaneous breathing still fails to occur, an attempt may be made if equipment is available to intubate the calf and provide positive pressure ventilation.

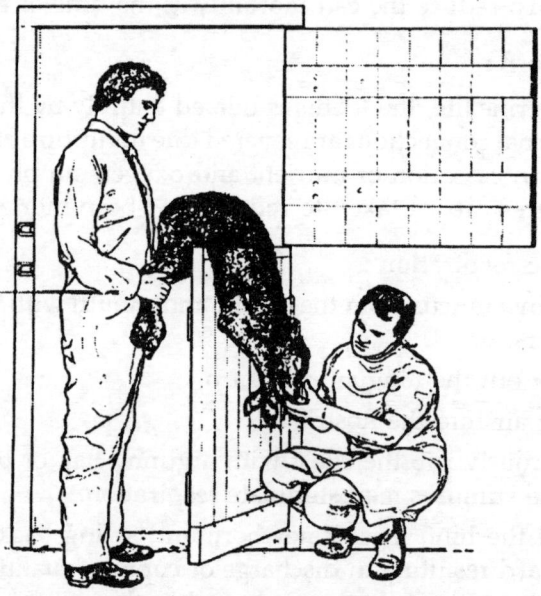

Fig. 17.1 : Resuscitation of the calf. Note that a calf is briefly suspended by its leg from a convenient beam or hung over a door. The chest is slapped gently to disloge the mucus.(Courtesy of Jackson, P.G.G. 1995. Handbook of Veternary Obstetrics. W. B. Saunders Company Limited.)

MOUTH TO MOUTH RESPIRATION

Mouth to mouth respiration should be avoided. Attempts to inflate the lungs by blowing through calf-nose or by using a mask will result in filling of air into the stomach, since the resistance to stomach inflation is less than the resistance to displacement of the lung fluid. Thus, this method is ineffective and also carries zoonotic risks.

- Once spontaneous breathing is established, the calf may be given further care. Severe dyspnoea may occur in immature calves and these animals should be given an intravenous injection of **2-4 mg. of dexamethasone** which encourages **surfactant production.**

INTERESTING FACTS

- The first breath marks the end of foetal life and the beginning of the postnatal period.
- In most cases, if resuscitation does not result in spontaneous respiration in 2 to 3 minutes, it is unlikely that the newborn will survive, even though there is a good strong pulse and heart beat.
- Maximum survival time of a calf without oxygen entering the lungs is 4-6 minutes.

---

2. **Prevention of umbilical infection :**

- If the umbilical cord is not ruptured, it should be ligated at about 2 inches from the umbilicus and severed with scissors, and the stump should be cleaned with antiseptic. **The navel cord should not be tied but allowed to drain if bleeding is not so profused.**
- To this stump, tincture iodine should be applied. The ligation should be removed within 12 - 24 hours.

3. **Thermo-regulation :**

Thermo-regulation in the newborn can be improved in a number of ways.

- Ensure that there is adequate milk intake.
- Arrange the birth to occur in a thermally neutral environment as far as possible.
- **New born puppy should be placed in an environmental temperature of 30-33°C for the first 24 hours, which can be reduced to 26-30°C by 3 days.**
- The new born's coat should be adequately and quickly dried.
- Suitable jacket should be provided in winter.

Note : **The new born has little subcutaneous fat and hence insulation is poor.**

4. **Management of acidosis :**

- The foetus at the time of a normal birth will usually have a mild metabolic and respiratory acidosis.
- Dystocia is likely to cause a severe respiratory and metabolic acidosis.

- Severe acidosis has an adverse effect on both respiratory and cardiac function.
- Signs of acidosis
  - Abdominal breathing.
  - Low heart rate.
  - Prolonged jugular filling time.
  - Poor body muscle tone.
  - Absence of a pedal reflex.
  - Time to attain sternal recumbency (T-SR) is greater than 15 minutes.

TSR of calf in different conditions :

Condition	T-SR
Unassisted delivery	4.0 ± 2.2 minutes.
Caesarean section	4.5 ± 3.1 minutes.
Assisted delivery	5.4 ± 3.3 minutes.
Severe traction	9.0 ± 3.5 minutes.

Note : *A T-SR of >15 minutes is an ominous sign of severe acidosis.*

- If there is no sign of spontaneous improvement, give 250-500 ml. of **4.2% sodium bicarbonate by slow intravenous injection.**

EFFECTS OF ACIDOSIS
- Poor colostrum uptake.
- Shortening of the period during which the calf is normally able to absorb antibodies.
- Abomasal atony.
- General dullness.
- Reluctance to move.
- Inability to suck the milk.

5. Colostrum feeding :

- The young one should get first colostrum within first two hours after birth.
- In case colostrum is not available, **200-500 ml. of dam's blood or serum** should be **injected subcutaneously to young one of large animal and in smaller animals, 20-100 ml.** to their young one (s) animal.

6.   Milk feeding :

The rate of milk feeding should be about 10% of the calf's weight per day upto a maximum of 5-6 litre/ day.

DO YOU KNOW ?

The domestic animal's new born differ in the selectivity and duration of their intestinal permeability. In horse and pig, protein absorption is selective, IgG and IgM are preferentially absorbed and IgA mainly remains in the intestine while in ruminants all classes of immunoglobulin are absorbed (i.e. non-selective).

7.   Regular vaccination.

8.   Dehorn the calf at an early age, preferably within 15 days.

9.   Inspection of natural orfices :

● The new-born should be examined carefully to ascertain that all the natural orifices are patent and if not, a timely surgical intervention is necessary.

10.   Retained meconium :

● The meconium may be retained. In such cases, the newborn shows colic symptoms and lack of appetite.

● The enema of saline, soap and water or glycerine or castor-oil should be given in this condition.

11.   Persistent urachus :

● It is characterized by **continuous dribbling of urine through urachus**.

● Cauterize the affected part with tincture iodine.

12.   Diseases of newborn :

White scour :

● It is caused by *E. coli* infection.

● It occurs very early in life or even in a day old calf.

● In acute cases, there is septicaemia and the calf is found dead.

● **Foetid diarrhoea, colour of faeces varies from yellowish brown to white.**

● Loss of appetite.

● Dehydration and sinking of eye.

- Treatment -
  - Withhold the milk
  - DNS – I/V
  - Antibiotics

Navel ill or Joint ill :
- In acute cases, death is sudden without any specific symptom.
- In less acute cases
  - Swelling of navel together with abscess formation.
  - Joints (especially back or knee) are usually hot, swollen and painful.
- Treatment – Antibiotics

Calf diphtheria :
- Caused by *Fusiformis necrophorus*.
- Swelling in the throat region.
- Laboured breathing.
- Coughing along with **sticky greenish discharge and the swollen tongue protrudes**.
- High mortality.
- Antibiotic therapy is indicated.

Calf pneumonia :
- Antibiotic therapy is indicated.

OBSERVATIONS :

Date : ....

- Case No. ....
- Species ....
- Weight of Newborn ....
- Pulse rate ....
- Temperature ....
- Respiration rate ....
- Effort to initiate respiration, if any   Yes/No.
- Type of effort (s) ....
- Result of effort (s) ....

- T-SR ....
- Jugular filling time ....
- Pedal reflex ....
- Meconium ....
- Micturation ....
- Colour and consistency of faeces ....
- Appetite ....
- Navel cord ....
- Percentage of dehydration ....
- Diagnosis ....
- **Treatment**
  Rx
  1.
  2.
  3.
  4.

EXERCISE :

1. In which species, retention of meconium is more common ?

Ans.

2. Why is the chest rubbed to initiate respiration in new born ?

Ans.

3. What is the effect of hanging the new born by its hind legs ?

Ans.

4. What is the doxapram chloride, write its dose and indications ?

Ans.

5. Why heat loss from the new born is more than from adult ?

Ans.

6. What is T-SR ?

Ans.

7. Write the signs of acidosis.

Ans.

8. Write the dose of sodium bicarbonate in the treatment of acidosis in a new born calf.

Ans.

9. What will happen, if excess pressure is given during compression of chest for artificial respiration of new born ?

Ans.

10. Why mouth to mouth respiration is not advocated ?

Ans.

11. Write the treatment of persistent urachus.

Ans.

✵ ✵ ✵ ✵ ✵

To handle yourself use your head; to handle others use your heart.

PART – II

OBSTETRICS

Special Features :

- It contains a lot of information along with photographs which are not generally given in any available routine text-book such as 'The Interesting Techniques of Vaginal Examination of a Bitch and Sow just before Parturition', 'Methods of Application of Calving Ropes', 'Protection of Uterine Wall from Sharp Teeth and Hoof' etc.

- Discussion of a new approach to caudal epidural anaesthesia in which xylazine or combination of xylazine and lignocaine is being used in place of lignocaine alone.

- Advantage and disadvantage of different operative sites for caesarean section.

- No detail discussion of each and every type of foetal disposition separately.

Chapter 18

Pelvices of Different Domestic Animals

Hip bones (Os coxae) : (See Fig. 18.1 and 18.2).

- There are two hip bones which form the bony pelvis.
- Each hip bone is formed by the **ilium, ischium** and **pubis**.

Ilium :

- It is a **triangular flat bone** situated at the cranio-lateral aspect of the pelvis.
- It has **two surfaces, three angles** and **three borders.**
- The broad, flat and dorsal part of the ilium is called wing.
- The medial portion (angle) of the wing is called tuber sacrale which articulates with the sacrum.
- The external portion (angle) of the wing is called **tuber coxae** or **'hook' bone.**
- The distal angle is narrow and considered as **shaft.**
- At the middle of the medial surface of the shaft, there is a raised prominence called **psoas tubercle.**
- The distal angle is expanded and joins ventrally with the ischium and pubis, and form **acetabulum.**
- The medial or pelvic surface of shaft is smooth and has groove for the obturator vessels and nerves.

Ischium :

- It is **quadrilateral in shape,** situated behind the pubis and forms most part of the pelvic floor.

- It has **two surfaces, four borders** and **four angles.**
- The **anterior border** is Concave and forms **posterior boundary of the obturator foramen.**
- The **posterior border** of an ischium joins with the posterior border of the opposite ischium and forms the **ischial arch.**

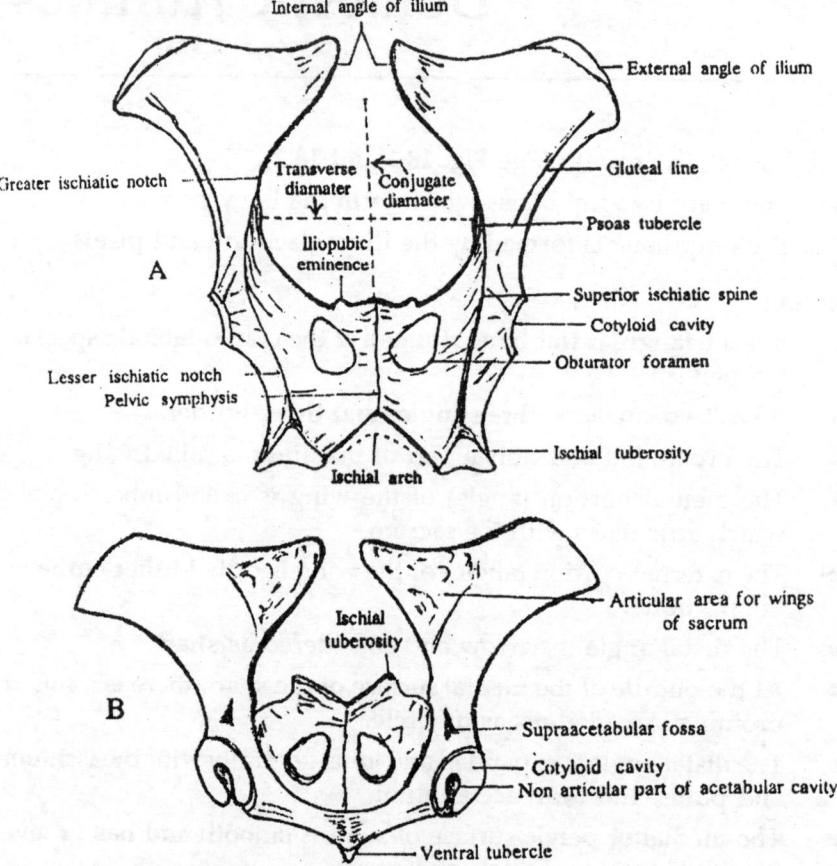

Fig. 18.1 : Hip bone of bovine (posterior view) B. Hip bone of bovine (anterior view)

- The **lateral border** forms the **lesser ischiatic notch.**
- The **medial border** of an ischium joins with the medial border of the opposite ischium and forms **ischial symphysis.**
- The antero-external angle joins with the cotyloid angles of ilium and pubis to form **cotyloid cavity (acetabulum).**
- The **posterio-external angle** forms ischial tuberosity or 'pin' bone.

96

Pubis :

- It is the **smallest of the three bones** of the os coxae (hip bone), which forms the cranial portion of the pelvic floor.

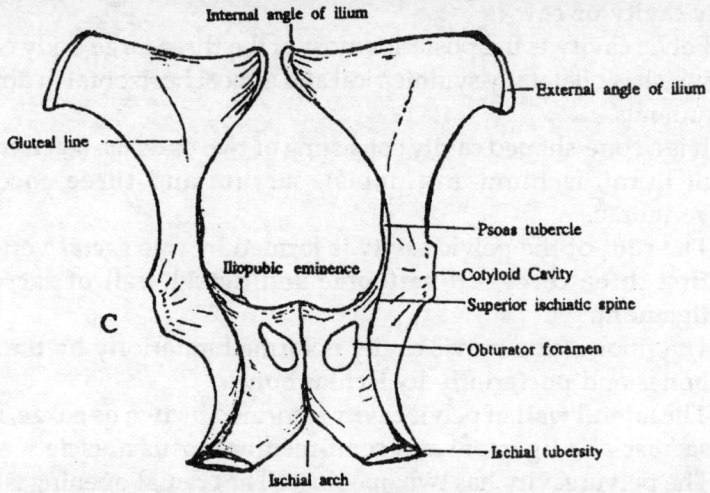

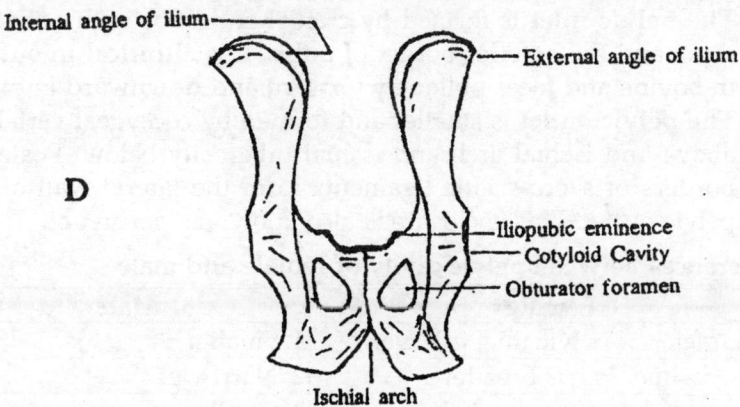

Fig. 18.2 : C. Hip bone of horse (posterior view) D. Hip bone of dog (posterior view). (Courtesy of Ghosh, R.K. 1995. Primary Veterinary Anatomy. Current Book International, for all figures of this chapter).

- The cranial medial border of the pubic bone provides attachment for the prepubic tendon.
- The caudal border forms the cranial border of the obturator foramen.
- The **medial border** of a pubis joins with the medial border of opposite pubis and forms **pubic symphysis.**

Obturator foramen :
- It is the **largest foramen** of the body.
- It is formed by the **ischium** and **pubis.**

Pelvic cavity of cow :
- Pelvic cavity is the posterior most of the three large body cavities which is bilaterally symmetrical and almost horizontal in domestic animals.
- It is a cone-shaped cavity consisting of two os coxae (each consists of ilium, ischium and pubis), **sacrum** and **three coccygeal vertebrae.**
- **The roof** of the pelvic cavity is formed by five **sacral vertebrae, first three coccygeal vertebrae** and **dorsal wall of sacro-iliac ligament.**
- The floor of the pelvic cavity is formed anteriorly by the **pubic bones** and **posteriorly by ischial bones.**
- **The lateral wall** of pelvic cavity is formed by **two os coxae, lateral sacrosciatic ligament** and **semi-membranosus muscle.**
- The pelvic cavity has two openings. The cranial opening is called **pelvic inlet** and caudal opening is called **pelvic outlet.**
- **The pelvic inlet** is formed by cranial end of sacrum, shaft of ilium and the anterior border of pubis. It is **elliptical in outline** in bovine and faces obliquely forward and downward in cattle.
- **The pelvic outlet** is smaller and formed by coccygeal vertebrae above and ischial arch and ischial tuberosity below. Posterior borders of sacro-sciatic ligaments form the lateral wall of the pelvic outlet. This enclosure is also known as **perineum.**

Differences between pelvic cavity of female and male

Female	Male
1. Diameter of pelvic inlet is larger	1. Smaller
2. The ischial arch is broader	2. Narrower
3. The obturator foramen is larger	3. Smaller
4. The floor of the cavity is wide & more concave	4. Narrow and less concave
5. The bones of pelvis are less thicker & heavier	5. Thicker & heavier
6. Pelvis is capacious	6. Less capacious

Pelvic cavity of mare :
- Transverse diameter and sacro-pubic diameter are nearly same.
- The tuber coxae are large and more prominent than those in cow.

- The wing of the ilium is nearly perpendicular to the long axis of the body.
- Pelvis is nearly round.

Pelvic cavity of ewe :

- The pelvic inlet is similar to that of cow in shape (elliptical).
- The wings are nearly parallel to each other.
- The ischial tuberosities are relatively much smaller than those in cow.

Pelvic cavity of sow :

- The pelvic inlet is long and narrow.
- The wings of the ilia are not prominent and large as in cow and mare.
- The pubic symphysis is thicker and does not undergo complete ankylosis.
- The ischial tuberosities are **not completely ossified.**

Pelvic cavity of bitch :

- The pelvic inlet is **oval in shape.**
- The wings of the ilia are small and nearly parallel to the vertebral column.
- The ischium is twisted in appearance.

Pelvic cavity of queen :

- The pelvis of the queen is similar to that of the bitch but has a relatively larger obturator foramen.

Pelvic ligament :

There are four pelvic ligaments (see Fig. 18.3) which also help in formation of pelvic cavity.

These are :

- Dorsal sacro-iliac ligament
- Lateral sacro-iliac ligament
- Ilio-lumbar ligament.
- Sacro-sciatic ligament.
- **The dorsal sacro-iliac ligament** extends from tuber sacrale to the summit of sacral spines in the form of a band.

- **The lateral sacro-iliac ligament** extends from tuber sacrale to the lateral border of sacrum.

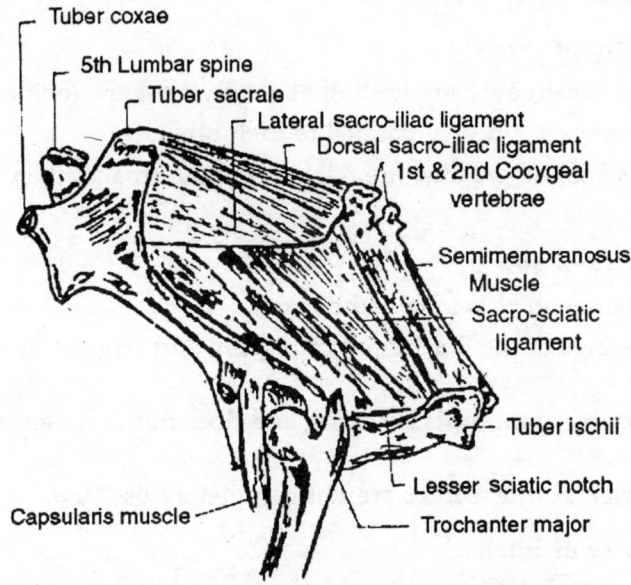

Fig. 18.3 : Diagram showing pelvic ligaments.

- **The ilio-lumbar ligament** extends from the transverse process of lumbar to the ventral surface of ilium.
- **The sacro-sciatic ligament** is an extensive quadrilateral ligamentous sheet that completes the lateral wall of the pelvic cavity. The ligament extends from the **lateral border of the sacrum** and the **transverse processes of the first two coccygeal** vertebrae to the **ischiatic spine and tuber ischii.**
- **The pre-pubic tendon** is essentially the **tendon of insertion of the recti abdominis muscle and other abdominal muscles except the transversus abdominis muscle.** It is attached strongly to the cranial border of the pubic bones. It maintains the bony pelvis in its proper position.

Thus, bones and ligaments form pelvic cavity.

Note : *The cow and sow have elliptical pelvic inlets while mare and bitch have round pelvic inlets.*

EXERCISE :

1. What is the difference between pelvic cavity of bitch and queen?

Ans.

2. When sacro-sciatic ligament become relaxed and why ?

Ans.

3. What is a 'hook' bone ?

Ans.

4. What is a 'pin' bone ?

Ans.

5. How is an acetabulum formed ?

Ans.

6. What is the shape of pelvic inlet of cow and sow ?

Ans.

7. What is the shape of pelvic inlet of mare and bitch ?

Ans.

8. Which species is more prone to rupture of prepubic tendon during pregnancy and why ?

Ans.

9. Which abdominal muscle is not inserted at prepubic tendon ?

Ans.

❊ ❊ ❊ ❊ ❊

Life's precious moments do not have value, unless they are shared.

Chapter 19

Pelvimetry of Domestic Animals

Study of pelvimetry is imperative because crossbreeding programme in our country is going on and foeto-pelvic disproportion is one of the major causes of dystocia.

Pelvimetry :

Pelvimetry is defined as branch of obstetrics which deals with measurement of the diameters of pelvis. The study of pelvimetry is very much desired for selective breeding and crossbreeding since the relationship between various diameters allow one to form an idea of shape, size, position of pelvis and the birth canal. It helps in culling of undesired animals which have narrow and defective pelvis. Pelvimetery in living animal is carried out in two ways viz.

1. **External/ indirect pelvimetry** : The calculation of different diameters of pelvis by certain measuremental device externally is called external pelvimetry.

2. **Internal/ direct pelvimetry** : The calculation of different diameters of pelvis by inserting hand through rectum and assessing different diameters by spans of thumb from index to middle finger and evenly spreading the little finger is called internal pelvimetry.

1. External/ indirect pelvimetry :

Procedure :

1. Measure the distance between the two angles of haunch i.e. external angle of ilium by placing a straight piece of wood vertically against each haunch and the distance between the two vertical wooden pieces is measured...................... (A)

2. Measure the distance between two ischial tuberosities directly. .... (B)

3. Measure the height from hip joint to the highest point of croup by placing a straight wooden piece horizontally across the summit of croup and the other straight wooden piece is put horizontally along the trochanter and the ischial tuberosity. The vertical distance in between the above two straight wooden pieces is the height from hip joint to the summit of croup. ....(C)

Calculation :

Pelvic outlet diameters :

Transverse diameter of the pelvic outlet (X) = 1/4 (A + B).

Superio-inferior diameter of the pelvic outlet (Y) = 3/4 C.

Pelvic inlet diameters :

Transverse or bis-iliac diameter of the pelvic inlet = 1.22 X.

Sacro-pubic diameter of the pelvic inlet = 1.3 Y.

2. Internal/ direct pelvimetry :

This is measured by direct manual examination of the interior of the pelvis. The distances between various parts of pelvis are measured by calibrated palms.

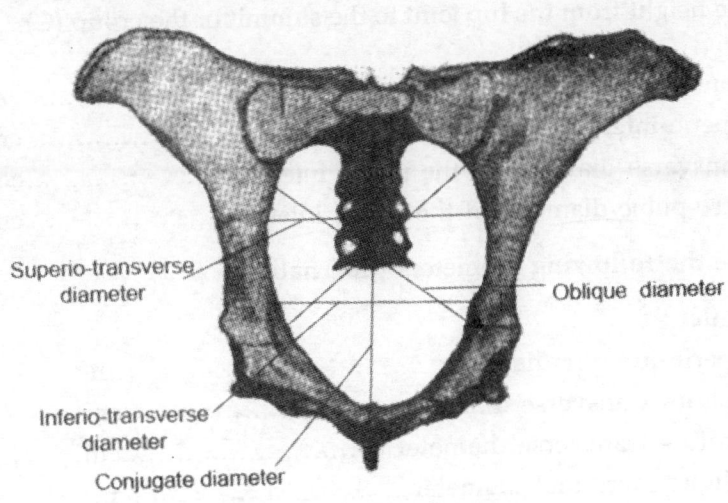

Superio-transverse diameter

Oblique diameter

Inferio-transverse diameter

Conjugate diameter

Fig. 19.1 : Diameters of Pelvic inlet

Diameters of pelvic inlet (see Fig. 19.1) :

1. **Superio-inferior or sacro-pubic or conjugate diameter** : It is measured from sacral promontory to the cranial end of the pubic symphysis.

2. **Superio-transverse diameter** : It is a transverse diameter at the greatest width i.e. **at upper third of the pelvic cavity.**

3. **Inferio-transverse diameter** : It is measured in lower fourth of pelvic cavity **between the two psoas tubercles.**

4. **Oblique sacro-ilial diameter** : It is measured from **sacroilial joint** through the centre of the pelvic cavity to **the psoas tubercle of the opposite side**.

5. **Vertical diameter** : It is measured from cranial end of the pubic symphysis to the junction of 3rd and 4th sacral verterbrae.

OBSERVATIONS :

Measure the following in cattle (externally) :

* Distance between the two angles of the haunch (A) ....cm.

* Distance between the two ischial tuberosities (B) ....cm.

* The height from the hip joint to the summit of the croup (C) ..... cm.

* Transverse diameter of the pelvic outlet (X) .... cm.

* Superio-inferior diameter of the pelvic outlet (Y) .... cm.

* Transverse diameter of the pelvic inlet ....cm.

* Sacro-pubic diameter of the pelvic inlet ....cm.

Measure the following diameters (internally):

Pelvic inlet :

* Superio-inferior diameter ....cm

* Superio- transverse diameter .... cm

* Inferio – transverse diameter ....cm

* Oblique sacro-ilial diameter ....cm

* Vertical diameter ....cm

Opinion :

Approximate pelvic diameters in different species (cm.) :

Species	Sacro-pubic	Transverse or bis-iliac
Mare	20.3 – 25.4	19.0 – 24.1
Cow	19.0 – 24.1	14.6 – 19.0
Sheep	7.6 – 10.8	5.7 – 8.9
Sow	9.5 – 15.2	6.3 – 10.2
Bitch	3.3 – 6.3	2.8 – 5.7

EXERCISE :

1. Define pelvimetry.

Ans.

2. What is pelvimeter ?

Ans.

3. Write the shape of pelvic inlet of different animals ?

Ans.

4. What is 'haunch' ?

Ans.

5. What is 'croup' ?

Ans.

�֎ ✷ ✷ ✷ ✷

Education is not something one acquires in the classroom. It begins the moment one is born and ends when one dies.

Chapter 20

Presentation, Position and Posture of Foetus

PRESENTATION : *It is relationship between longitudinal axis of dam with the longitudinal axis of foetus and parts present towards birth canal.* The presentation may be divided into three parts :

    (i)   Longitudinal presentation (normal).

    (ii)   Transverse presentation (abnormal).

    (iii)   Vertical presentation (abnormal).

(i) **Longitudinal presentation :** When longitudinal axis of dam is parallel to the longitudinal axis of vertebral column of foetus, the presentation is called longitudinal presentation. It is of two types :

    (a) **Anterior longitudinal presentation :** When foetus is in longitudinal presentation and its anteriormost parts i.e. both fore limbs and head are present towards birth canal, the presentation is called anterior longitudinal presentation (see Fig. 20.1).

    (b) **Posterior longitudinal presentation :** When foetus is in longitudinal presentation and posterior parts of the foetus i.e. both hind limbs are present towards birth canal, the presentation is called posterior longitudinal presentation (see Fig. 20.2).

(ii) **Transverse presentation :** When longitudinal axis of foetus forms a **right angle** with the long axis of dam **in transverse plane,** the presentationis is called as transverse presentation. It is of three types :

    (a) **Dorso-transverse or dorso-lumbar :** When longitudinal axis of foetus forms a right angle with the long axis of dam in transverse plane and dorsum (vertebral column) of the foetus becomes convex and faces the pelvic inlet, the condition is called dorso-transverse presentation (see Fig. 20.3) or when

106

foetus is in transverse presentation and its dorsum faces the pelvic inlet, the presentation is called dorso-transverse presentation.

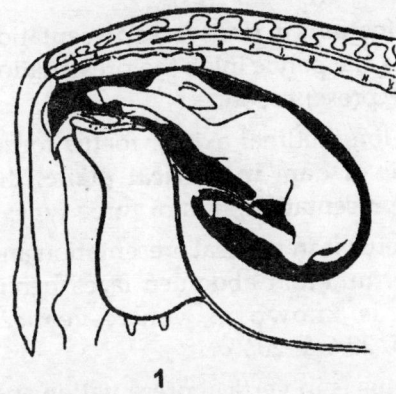

Fig. 20.1 : Normal anterior presentation.

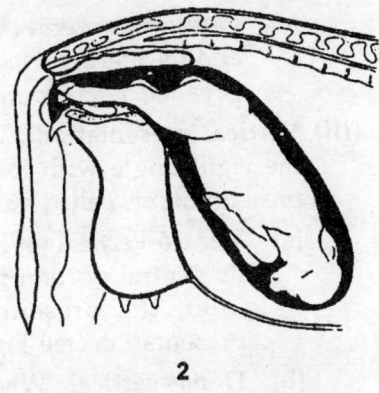

Fig. 20.2 : Posterior presentation.

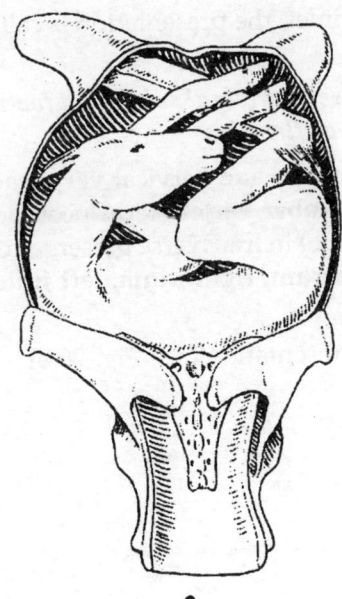

Fig. 20.3 : Dorso-transverse presentation in the mare.

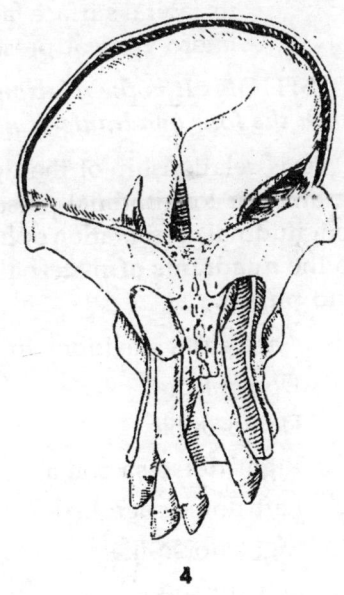

Fig. 20.4 : Ventro-transverse presentation in the mare.

(b) **Ventro-transverse or sterno-abdominal :** When foetus is in transverse presentation and its ventral or sterno-abdominal surface faces the pelvic inlet, the presentation is called ventro transverse presentation (see Fig. 20.4).

(c) **Latero-transverse :** When foetus is in transverse presentation and its lateral surface faces the pelvic inlet, the presentation is called latero-transverse presentation.

(iii) **Vertical presentation :** When longitudinal axis of foetus forms the right angle with long axis of dam **in vertical plane,** the presentation is called vertical presentation. It is of three types :

(a) **Ventro-vertical :** When foetus is in vertical presentation and its ventral portion i.e. sternum and abdomen faces pelvic inlet, the presentation is known as ventro-vertical presentation (see Fig. 20.5, 20.6 & 20.7).

(b) **Dorso-vertical :** When foetus is in vertical presentation and its dorsum (i.e. vertebral column) faces pelvic inlet, the presentation is called dorso-vertical presentation.

(c) **Latero-vertical :** When foetus is in vertical presentation and its lateral surface faces pelvic inlet, the presentation is called latero-vertical presentation.

POSITION : *It is the relationship between vertebral column of foetus with the four quadrants of pelvic inlet of the dam.*

Or It is relationship of the **dorsum** (thoracic and cervical vertebrae) in anterior longitudinal presentation, **lumbar vertebrae** in posterior longitudinal presentation or **head (cephalo)** in transverse presentation to the **quadrants of maternal pelvis (sacrum, right ilium, left ilium and pubis).**

There are **eight positions** in anterior presentation (see Fig. 20.5).

1. Dorso-sacral.
2. Dorso-pubic.
3. Right dorso-sacroilial.
4. Left dorso-sacroilial.
5. Right dorso-ilial.
6. Left dorso-ilial.
7. Right dorso-supra cotyloid.
8. Left dorso-supra cotyloid.

There are **eight positions** in posterior presentation (see Fig 20.6):

1. Lumbo-sacral.

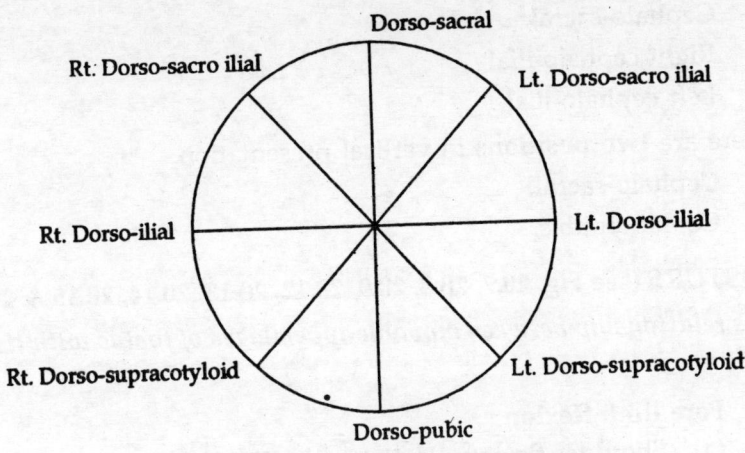

Fig. 20.5 : Positions in anterior presentation.

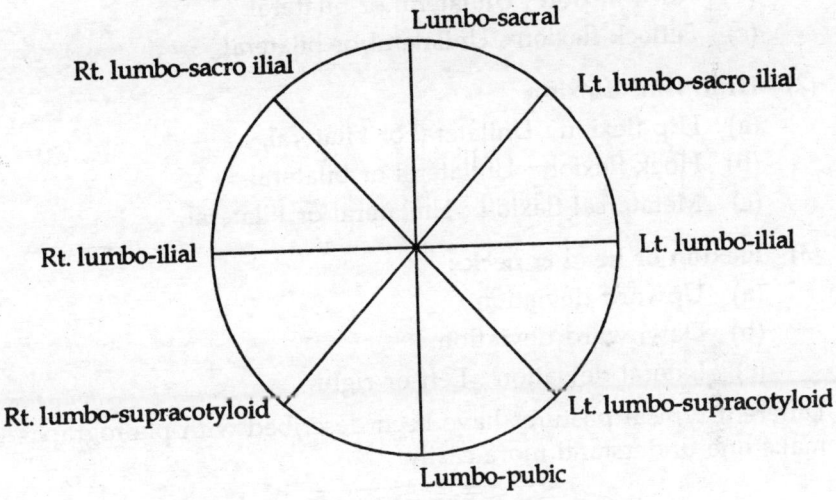

Fig. 20.6 : Positions in posterior presentation.

2. Lumbo-pubic.
3. Right lumbo-sacroilial.
4. Left lumbo-sacroilial.
5. Right lumboilial.
6. Left lumboilial.
7. Right lumbo-supra cotyloid.
8. Left lumbo-supra cotyloid.

There are **six positions** in transverse presentation (three each in dorso-lumbar and sterno- abdominal).

1.   Cephalo-sacral.
2.   Right cephalo-ilial.
3.   Left cephalo-ilial.

There are **two positions** in vertical presentation.
1.   Cephalo-sacral.
2.   Cephalo-pubic.

POSTURE (see Fig. 20.7, 20.8, 20.9, 20.12, 20.13, 20.14, 20.15 & 20.16):
It is relationship between movable appendages of foetus with its own body.

(1) Fore limb flexion :
   (a) Shoulder flexion : Unilateral or bilateral.
   (b) Knee flexion : Unilateral or bilateral.
   (c) Fetlock flexion : Unilateral or bilateral.

(2) Hind limb flexion :
   (a) Hip flexion : Unilateral or bilateral.
   (b) Hock flexion : Unilateral or bilateral.
   (c) Metatarsal flexion : Unilateral or bilateral.

(3) Flexion of head & neck :
   (a) Upward deviation.
   (b) Downward deviation.
   (c) Lateral deviation : Left or right.

Different typical postures have been described with photographs to make one understand more easily.

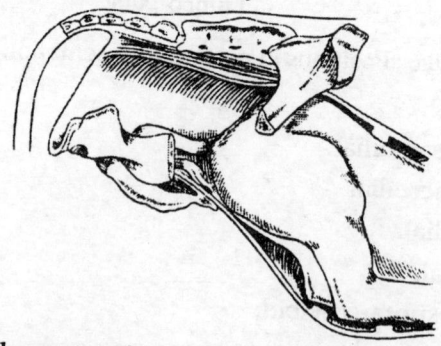

Fig. 20.7 : Breech presentation : Posterior presentation, dorso-sacral position and bilaterla hip flexion posture. (Courtesy of Noakes, D.E., Parkinson, J.T. and Egland, G.C.W. 2001. Arthur's Veterinary Reproducion and Obstetrics).

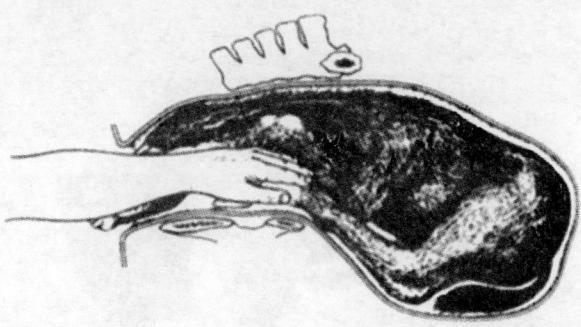

Fig. 20.8 : Foal in 'dog-sitting position'. Presentation-oblique ventro-vertical, Position-dorsosacral and Posture-dog sitting. (Courtesy of Benesch, F. and Wright, J.G. 2001. Veterinary obstetrics. Greenworld Publishers).

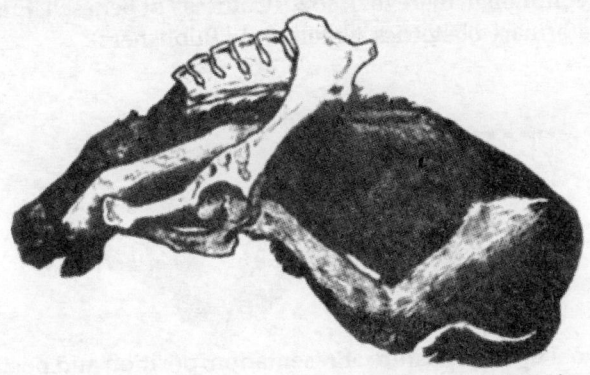

Fig. 20.9 : Ventro-vertical presentation (Dog-sitting position) with anterior end of body still lying in the pelvis. (Courtesy of Benesch, F. and Wright, J.G. 2001. Veterinary obstetrics. Greenworld Publishers).

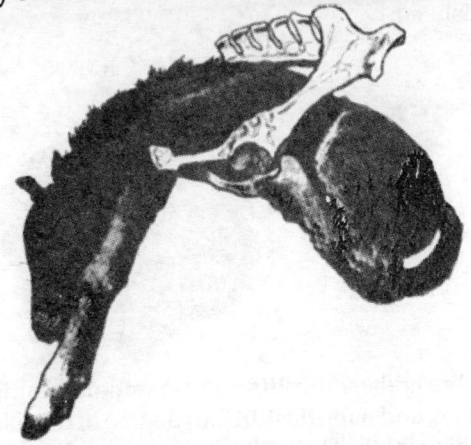

Fig. 20.10 : Ventro-vertical presentation (Dog-sitting position) partially delivered. (Courtesy of Benesch, F. and Wright, J.G. 2001. Veterinary obstetrics. Greenworld Publishers).

111

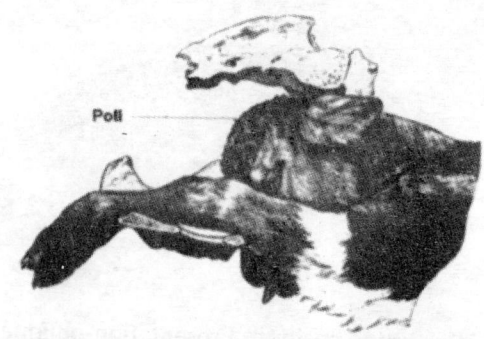

Fig. 20.11 : Foal in vertex posture : Presentation-anterior, Position-dorso sacral, Posture-downward displacement of head and poll is directed into pelvic inlet. More common in mare than cow. (Courtesy of Benesch, F. and Wright, J.G. 2001. Veterinary obstetrics. Greenworld Publishers).

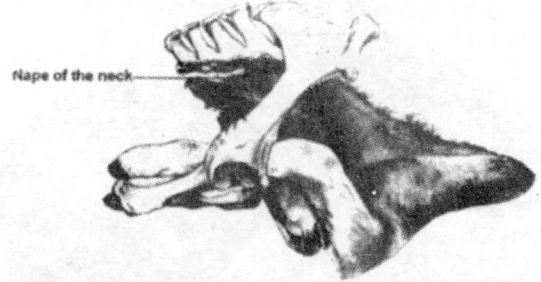

Fig. 20.12 : Foal in nape posture : Presentation, position and posture are the same as vertex posture but degree of downward displacement of head is more so that part of the nape of the neck is directed towards the pelvic inlet. (Courtesy of Benesch, F. and Wright, J.G. 2001. Veterinary obstetrics. Greenworld Publishers).

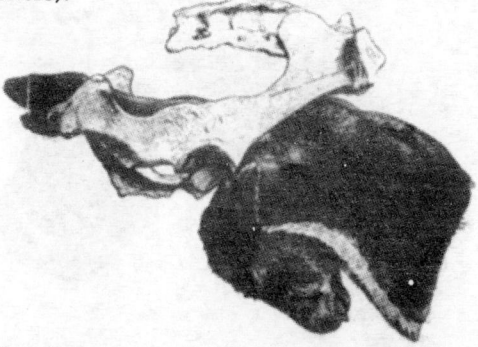

Fig. 20.13 : Foal in breast-head posture : Presentation, position and posture are the same as vertex and nape posture but degree of displacement of head is more than the above both. The ventrally flexed neck is situated between the forelimbs, the jaw being adjacent to the sterum. (Courtesy of Benesch, F. and Wright, J.G. 2001. Veterinary obstetrics. Greenworld Publishers).

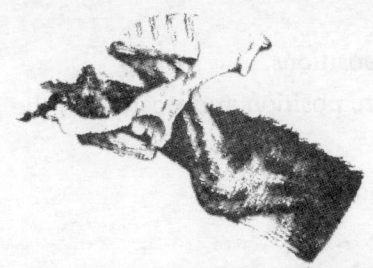

Fig. 20.14 : Foot nape posture (bilateral) : Presentation-anterior, Position-dorsosacral, Posture-upward deviation of both forelimbs. This defect is peculiar in the foal because of its cylindrical neck and longer limbs. (Courtesy of Benesch, F. and Wright, J.G. 2001. Veterinary obstetrics. Greenworld Publishers).

IMPORTANT POINTS
• The normal presentation in a uniparous animal is the anterior longitudinal presentation, dorso-sacral position with the head resting on the metacarpal bones and knees of the extended forelegs.
• Birth can take place without assistance, if the foetus is in the posterior longitudinal presentation and lumbo-sacral position.
• The transverse presentation is seen only rarely in ruminants and multipara.
• The transverse presentation can occur in the mare in which the foetus develops in both the uterine horns rather than the uterine body and one horn.
• Posterior longitudinal presentation in a multiparous animal is considered normal or physiological.
• Posture in multiparous animal is of no importance because their limbs are small, short and flexible.

Commonest cause of dystocia in different animals :	
• Cow	- Foetomaternal disproportion
• Mare	- Lateral deviation of head
• Ewe & doe	- * Foetomaternal disproportion
	* Among maldisposition – shoulder flexion
• Sow	- Primary uterine inertia
• Bitch	- Primary uterine inertia

EXERCISE :

1. Define foetal dispositions.
2. Write presentation, position and posture of the following foetal dispositions.

(a) Breech presentation :

Presentation ....

Position ....

Posture ....

(b) Dog-sitting position :

Presentation ....

Position ....

Posture ....

(c) Foot nape posture

Presentation ....

Position ....

Posture ....

(d) Butt or poll or vertex posture

Presentation ....

Position ....

Posture ....

(e) Nape posture

Presentation ....

Position ....

Posture ....

(f) True breast-head posture

Presentation ....

Position ....

Posture ....

4   Write the most common foetal maldisposition in the following species :

(a) Cow ....

(b) Ewe ....

(c) Doe ....

(d) Sow ....

(e) Mare ....

(f) Bitch ....

(g) Queen ....

❈ ❈ ❈ ❈ ❈

On earth there is nothing great but man; in man there is nothing great but mind.   *– S.W. Hamilton.*

Chapter 21

Caudal Epidural Anaesthesia

Epidural anaesthesia :

When a local anaesthetic agent is given between the space formed by endosteum and duramater such an anaesthesia is known as epidural anaesthesia.

Site for epidural anaesthesia :

Cattle & Buffalo	:	Last sacral and first coccygeal vertebrae or in between 1st and 2nd coccygeal vertebrae.
Equine	:	Between 1st & 2nd coccygeal vertebrae.
Sheep and goat	:	Same as cattle.
Pig and dog	:	Last lumbar & first sacral vertebrae.

MECHANISM OF ACTION

- Epidural injection is a **nerve block, not a spinal anaesthesia** because the injection is given outside the duramater after the end of the spinal cord. Spinal cord containing the spinal fluid, terminates between the second to fourth sacral vertebrae in the cow and the first to third sacral vertebrae in the mare. Therefore, at the site of caudal epidural anaesthesia, there is no spinal fluid present (Fig. 21.2).
- Thus, it is a form of multiple spinal nerve block in which **the coccygeal** and **posterior sacral nerves are desensitized..**
- These nerves supplied to the **anus, perineum, vulva** and **vagina** only.

Technique of epidural injection :

- The site is clipped and thoroughly washed with an antiseptic solution and the sacro-coccygeal region is shaved.
- The exact site is located by holding the tail below the base and moving it upward and downward in a **pump handle fashion.**
- Now bring the thumb of left hand near the sacro-coccygeal region

and feel the depression between the last sacral and 1st coccygeal vertebrae. The site of sacro-coccygeal is easily palpable because sacrum remains fixed whereas first coccygeal vertebra moves.

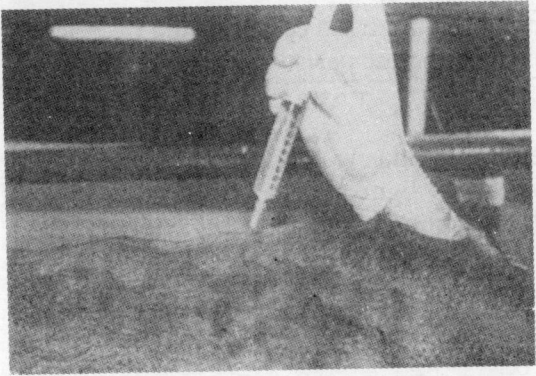

Fig. 21.1 : Site of injection of caudal epidural anaesthesia in adult cattle is the inter-vertebral space between the first and second coccygeal vertebrae.

- Desensitize the skin over the injection site by injecting small volume of local anaesthetic.

  Hold the needle (16 gauze and 5 cm. long) and insert into the above site at about 90^0 in cattle and in case of mare, 1st and 2nd coccygeal space at **about 45⁰ angle (See Fig. 21.1).**
- When needle pierces endosteum, there will be **crackling sound** which indicates that the needle has crossed endosteum.
- Deposit the required amount of local anaestheti (lignocaine) and remove the needle carefully.

INTERESTING FACTS
• To confirm that the needle is correctly placed or not, attach the syringe to needle and make a trial injection, *if there is no resistance to flow of anaesthetic solution that means the needle point is in the epidural space.*
• Other method to know the correct placement of needle is, to put a few drops of local anaesthetic in the hub of the needle. When needle is in correct position, the anaesthetic solution will be sucked as a result of the negative pressure which exist inside.

117

NOTE :

- Within 2 minutes of injection, **the tail becomes flaccid and** in 10-20 minutes perineum gets desensitized as well as straining reflex is completely abolished.

- Induction of anaesthesia can be tested by pricking the needle in different dependent parts.

Drugs and doses :

- A heifer and small cow require a volume of **5 ml.** and **large cows 7-10 ml.** of 2% lignocaine hydrochloride to produce obstetric anaesthesia lasting about **30-150 minutes.**

Site of epidural anaesthesia

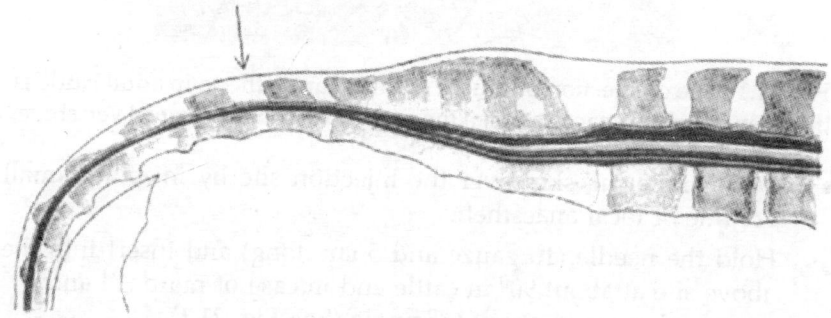

Fig. 21.2 : Diagram to demostrate the spinal meninges and the distribution of the space in the vertebral canal of the cow (Region of the os sacrum). Note that at the site of caudal epidural anaesthesia, there is no spinal fluid present. (Courtesy of Benesch, F. and Wright, J.G. 2001. Veterinary obstetrics. Greenworld Publishers).

- If 2% adrenaline is added, it prolongs the period of anaesthesia.
- In adult sheep and goat, approximately 2 ml. of 2% lignocaine induce sperineal anaesthesia.
- In sheep and goat 3 ml. of 2% lignocaine may cause **ataxia** and **recumbency.**
- In general, use of higher dose than recommended cause **hind limb incordination and sternal recumbency.**

CLINICAL POINTERS

- Continuous caudal epidural anaesthesia can be given to the cattle and small ruminants for giving relief from tenesmus caused by *chronic rectal or vaginal prolapse*. For this, place an 18-gauze & 5-cm long spinal catheter in the epidural space, remove the stylet, then place a catheter adapter on the hub of the catheter and secure the catheter to the skin. After securing the catheter in the skin, administer 3 to 5ml. of 2 % lignocaine every 1 to 3 hours or as needed.
- Bupivacaine is a safer, long-acting agent for epidural anaesthesia that provides analgesia for 4 to 6 hours after a single injection. The dose is the same as for 2% lignocaine hydrochloride.
- Administration of alcohol for long term epidural anaesthesia causes demyelination of nerves. This damage may extend to the sciatic nerve root, resulting in long-lasting or permanent effects and even rear-limb paralysis may occur. Therefore, use of alcohol for epidural anaesthesia is not recommended.

Advantages :

- Because epidural anaesthesia densensitizes anus, perineum, vulva and vagina, it resulting in **painless birth.**
- Outstanding advantage of epidural anaesthesia for an obstetrician is that it abolishes pelvic sensation reflex (pain) and abdominal contraction (straining), thus foetal manipulation and retropulsion becomes easier and defaecation remains suspended.
- If animal is recumbent due to pain, it often gets up after administration of epidural anaesthetic because painful pelvic sensation is abolished. This again makes the obstetrician's task easy because the manipulation in standing condition is easy.
- The epidural anaesthesia is useful whenever straining is vigorous as in prolapse of the uterus, vagina, rectum or urinary bladder.

Myometrial contraction and straining

Presence of foetus in the cervix and vagina leads to initiation of Fergusson's reflex and initiation of pelvic reflex. Fergusson's reflex causes stronger myometrial contractions while **pelvic reflex** leads to **strong abdominal contractions or straining.** The pelvic reflex is similar to that of defaecation reflex.

IMPORTANT POINTS

- *It should be clearly kept in mind that epidural anaesthesia does not inhibit myometrial contraction; it has no effect on the third stage of labour or uterine involution, because many veterinarians think that it reduces the myometrial contraction.*
- *With proper epidural anaesthesia, the animal stands quietly without moving or lying down, which is helpful to the operator.*
- *When it is used in caesarean section, it controls straining and prevents intestinal prolapse through the operative site.*
- *It may prevent prolapse of the uterus immediately after a difficult parturition because it reduces straining.*
- *Epidural anaesthesia in sheep and goat is not practical but seldom used because the abdominal contractions are not strong enough to interfere greatly with manual manipulations of the foetus.*

Indications :

- Correction of maldisposition of foetus
- Vulvar suture
- Prolapse of vagina, uterus, anus and urinary bladder
- Episiotomy
- Foetotomy
- Caesarean section
- Retention of foetal membrane

DO YOU KNOW ?

- *In recent years, 2% xylazine solution (0.05 to 0.12 mg/kg of body weight) diluted to a volume of 5 to 12 ml with 0.9% sterile saline has been used for epidural injection in place of lignocaine.*
- *The onset of perineal anaesthesia with xylazine within 10 to 20 minutes and duration of epidural anaesthesia is 3 to 4 hours.*
- *Thus xylazine-induced analgesia lasts longer than 2% lignocaine.*
- *Xylazine in combination with lignocaine may also be used for epidural anaesthesia in cattle.*
- *The recommended doses for 450 kg. cattle are 0.03 mg/kg of xylazine added to 2% lignocaine hydrochloride to a total volume of 5 ml.*
- *The combination of xylazine and lignocaine provides a longer duration of analgesia (about 4 to 5 hours).*

Epidural anaesthesia in mare :

Lignocaine	Xylazine
1. More ataxia	1. Less ataxia
2. Onset is rapid (approx. 5 min.)	2. Onset is slow (approx. 30 min.)
3. Duration of analgesia short (approx. 20 min.)	3. Duration of analgesia longer (approx. 210 min.)

NOTE : A combination of xylazine (0.17 mg/kg) and lignocaine (0.22 mg/ kg) can also be administered with rapid onset (approx. 5 min.) and prolonged duration of anaesthesia (approx. 330 min.) with minor signs of ataxia in mares.

Terminology used in epidural anaesthesia :

(i) High epidural anaesthesia : It is given at lumbo-sacral region i.e. between the last lumber and the first sacral vertebrae.

(ii) Low epidural anaesthesia :

It is given between the last sacral and first coccygeal or between the first and second coccygeal vertebrae depending upon the species. The low epidural anaesthesia is further subdivided into two, based on the doses of anaesthesia.

(a) Anterior epidural anaesthesia-**High doses of local anaesthetic are required.**

(b) Posterior epidural anaesthesia – **Low doses of local anaesthetic are required.**

IMPORTANT POINT
During the puncture of the epidural space, sometimes artery or vein is punctured and blood escapes. In this condition, the anaesthetic solution can still be injected without any harm or if necessary, the needle can be withdrawn, the clot cleaned and re-inserted.

OBSERVATIONS :

Date ....

- Case No. ....
- Species ....
- Age ....
- History of animal ....
- Site of epidural anaesthesia ....
- Name of local anaesthetic ....

- Dose ....
- Time required for tail to become flaccid .... minutes.
- Duration of analgesia ....minutes.

EXERCISE :

1. When does crackling sound come during the administration of epidural anaesthesia ?

Ans.

2. How will you confirm that the needle is in the epidural space ?

Ans.

3. How much time will be required for tail to become flaccid after giving epidural anaesthesia ?

Ans.

4. What is the dose of lignocaine to produce obstetrical anaesthesia ?

Ans.

5. What will happen, if lignocaine is administered at a higher dose than its recommended dose ?

Ans.

6. Xylazine is an analgesic, sedative and skeletal muscle relaxant. Can it be used in place of lignocaine in epidural anaesthesia?

Ans.

7. Write duration of analgesia of lignocaine, xylazine and combination of lignocaine and xylazine.

Ans.

8. Which drug is used to counteract side-effects of xylazine and write its dose.

Ans.

9. How will you manage the case of chronic rectal or vaginal prolapse by using epidural anaesthesia ?

Ans.

10. What are the side-effects of using alcohol in place of lignocaine in inducing epidural anaesthesia ?

Ans.

11. How can epidural anaesthesia help in retention of lubricant inside the uterus ?

Ans.

12. Why a recumbent animal due to malhandling of dystocia gets up after administration of epidural anaesthesia ?

Ans.

> *A single conversation across the table with a wise man is worth a month's study of books.*

Chapter 22

Obstetrical Instruments

Obstetrical instruments are grouped into various categories namely.

A. Instruments used for traction or extraction of foetus.

B. Instruments used for incising or excising.

C. Instruments used for repulsion and rotation.

D. Instruments used in foetotomy.

E. Miscellaneous equipment.

A. Instruments used for traction :

*   **Ropes** – Made of nylon or cotton. It has a loop on one end and the other end is loopless.

*   **Chains** - Obstetrical chains are made up of metal.

*   **Wooden handle** – It is about a foot in length.

*   **Whelping forceps** : It is used to apply traction in small animals like bitches and does.

*   **Hooks** : Hooks are used to hold the foetal parts where hand cannot reach and surfaces are slippery (see Fig. 22.1).

*   **Krey Schottler's hook** (multi-joint traction hook). This hook has 4 hinge joints (movable joints) with a movable ring. This is used for force traction of **dead foetus**. It is placed in **head or eye-ball**. During traction, its hooks enter the tissues of foetus and avoid laceration of the birth canal.

*   **Harris eye hook** : The hook is used for traction of the **dead foetus**. The hook is inserted behind the incision or in the **inner canthus of eye.**

*   **Obermayer's anal hook** : It consists of a long handle and an eye on one side and hook on other side. It is used at time of **breech presentation and** inserted in anus or at croup region for extraction of foetus.

*   **Robert's hook** – used for traction of the **dead foetus.**

- **Freyburger's hook :** This is used for traction of **live foetus**. These hooks have three parts viz. **hook proper, handle** and **eye for passing ropes**. After passing the rope, hooks are attached behind orbital fossa and the foetus is pulled outside.

Classification

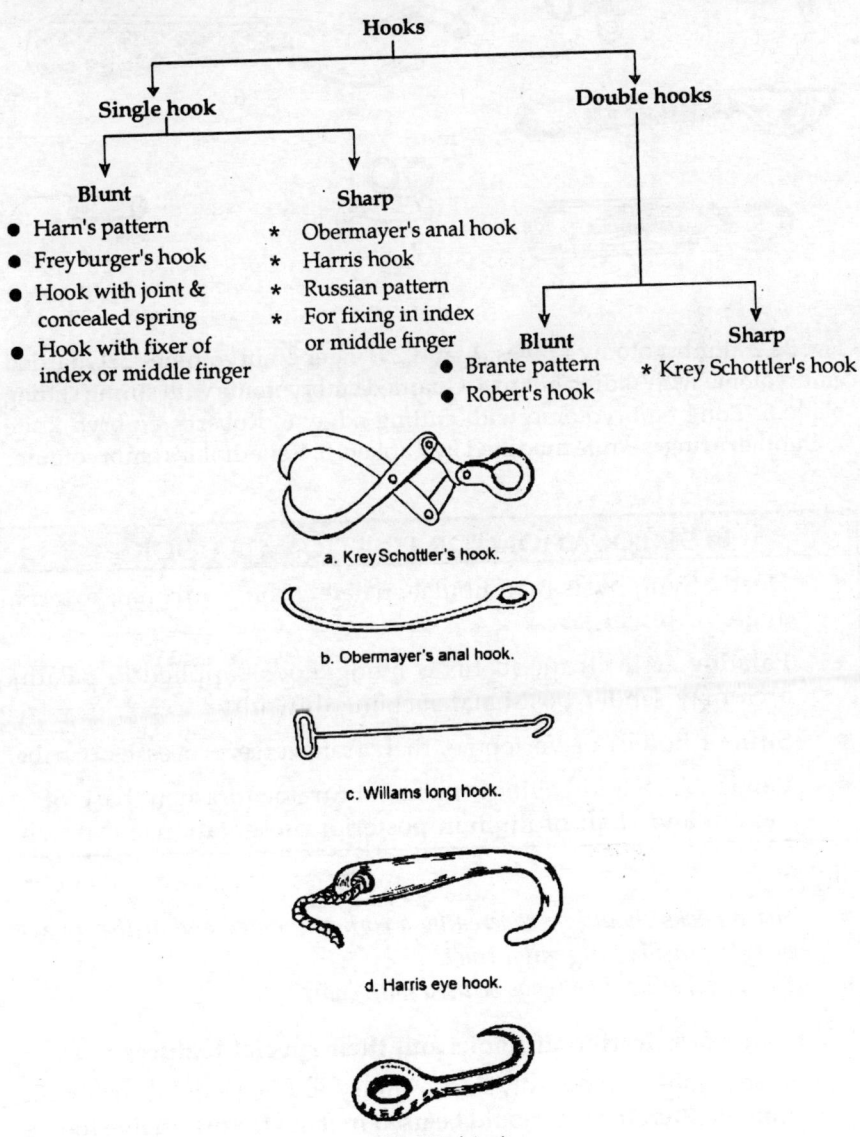

```
                        Hooks
           ┌──────────────┴──────────────┐
      Single hook                    Double hooks
    ┌─────────┴─────────┐                 │
  Blunt             Sharp                 │
```

Single hook

Blunt
- Harn's pattern
- Freyburger's hook
- Hook with joint & concealed spring
- Hook with fixer of index or middle finger

Sharp
* Obermayer's anal hook
* Harris hook
* Russian pattern
* For fixing in index or middle finger

Double hooks

Blunt
- Brante pattern
- Robert's hook

Sharp
* Krey Schottler's hook

a. Krey Schottler's hook.

b. Obermayer's anal hook.

c. Willams long hook.

d. Harris eye hook.

e. Short blunt hook.

Fig. 22.1 : Showing different types of hooks.

125

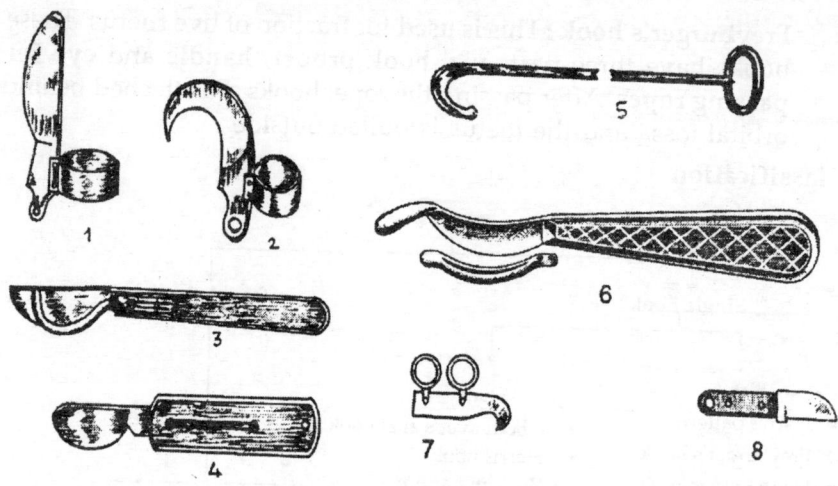

Fig. 22.2 : Embryotomy knives. 1. and 2. Finger embryotomes 3. Guarded embryotome with sliding guard 4. Guarded embryotome with spring sliding blade 5. Long embryotome with cutting edge. 6. Robert's embryo knife 7. Gunther's finger-knife modified by Tapken. 8. Venerholm's embryotome.

BEST LOCATION FOR FIXATION OF HOOKS

- **Head** : Symphysis mandibulae, palate, orbit, ear canal, **external angle of lower jaw.**

- **Palatine arch** : If the foetus is living, hooks applied to palatine arch may render post-natal suckling difficulty.

- **Spine** : Bodies of vertebrae, their transverse processes or ribs.

- **Pelvis** : Cotyloid cavities, pubis, obturator foramen, base of sacrum and shaft of ilium in posterior presentation.

NOTE :
- *Sharp hooks should be covered by a cork at pointed end at the time of carrying inside the genital tract.*
- *Short hooks should always be used with snare.*

Different classification of hooks and their special features :
- **Sharp hooks** frequently cause injury either to operator or the animal. Therefore, it should be used in **dead foetus.** In live foetus, mostly **blunt hooks** are used.

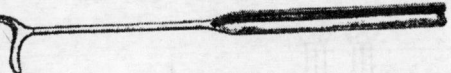

Fig. 22.3 : Keller's semisharp spatula. It is especially useful for decortication of limb and subsequent division of muscles attached to the trunk

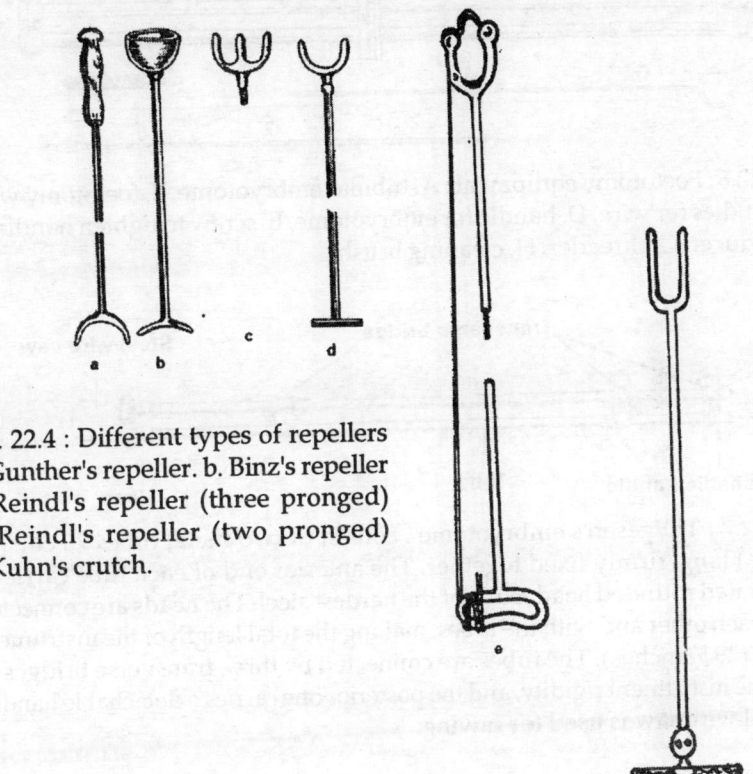

Fig. 22.4 : Different types of repellers
a. Gunther's repeller. b. Binz's repeller
c. Reindl's repeller (three pronged)
d. Reindl's repeller (two pronged)
e. Kuhn's crutch.

Fig. 22.5 : Cammerer's torsion tork

- **Short hooks** have an **eye** on one end through which cords run while long hooks have **handle** to operate. Hence **long hooks are easy to handle from outside.**

- The hooks are further classified as eye hook and anal hook. The **eye hooks** are applied at the **inner canthus of the eye** for traction whereas the **anal hooks** are applied at the **pubis.** Anal hooks are slightly longer than the eye hooks.

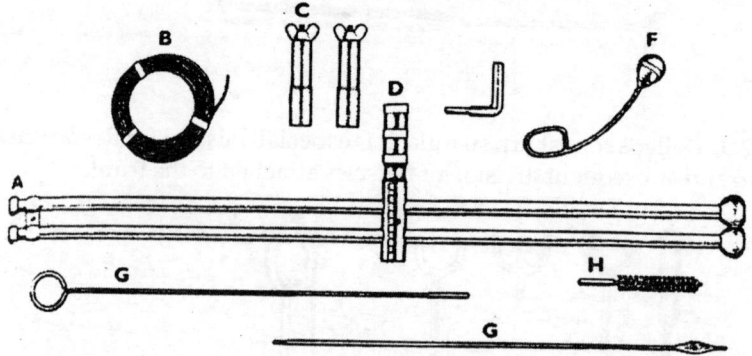

Fig. 22.6 : Foetotomy equipment : A. tubular embryotome, B. foetotomy wire, C. handles for wire, D. handle for embryotome, E. screw to tighten handle, F. introducer, G. threader, H. cleaning brush.

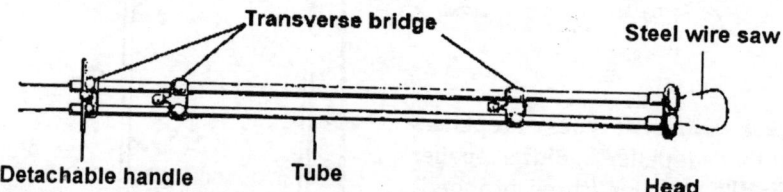

Fig. 22.7 : Thygesen's embryotome : consist of two metal tubes 70 cm. (28 inches) long, firmly fixed together. The anterior end of each tube carries a perforated rounded head made of the hardest steel. The heads are connected with each other and with the tubes, making the total length of the instrument 73 cm (29 ½ inches). The tubes are connected by three transverse bridges to give the instrument rigidity, and the posterior one carries a detachable handle. A steel wire saw is used for sawing.

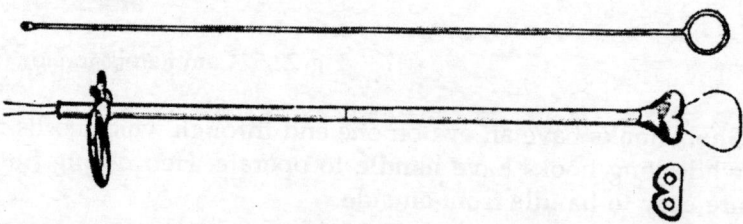

Fig. 22.8 : Neubarth's foetotome. This comprises a single metal tube, 75 cm (30 inches) long, made in two parts and connected by a screw joint. The head is screwed on the shaft. The total length of the instrument, with head is 80 cm. (32 inches).

B. Instruments used for incision and excision (see Fig. 22.2):

1. Finger embryotomes
2. Guarded embryotome with sliding guard
3. Guarded embryotome with spring sliding blade
4. Long embryotome with cutting edge
5. Robert's embryotomy knife
6. Gunther's finger knife modified by Tapken
7. Venerholm's embryotome

- **Chisel :** It is used for separating skin during abdominal and thoracic evisceration and it is also used in emphysematous foetus.
- **Spatula :** For **subcutaneous embryotomy,** Keller's semi-sharp spatula is most commonly used (see Fig. 22.3).

C. Instruments used for retropulsion & rotation :

Repeller :
- Kuhn's crutch
- Gunther's repeller
- Binz's repeller
- Reindl's repeller.

Rotator : (see Fig. 22.5)
- Cornell's detorsion rod.
- **Cammerer's torsion fork.**

D. Foetotome (see Figs. 22.6, 22.7 & 22.8) :

- There are many types of foetotome like Neubarth's foetotome, Thygesen's foetotome etc.
- The Thygesen's foetotome is the most commonly used foetotome. It has **two steel tubes** 70 cm (28 inch) in length and kept together by means of **a stay.** There is a **round head** on one end and **a holding hand** on the other end. A steel saw wire is passed through the tubes to form a desired size of loop at the anterior end. Both the ends of saw wire are fixed with metal handles separately.
- The heads are connected with each anterior end of tubes, making the total length of the instrument 73 cm (29.5 inches).

E. Miscellaneous Equipment :

Buckets, soap, several types of antiseptics, common surgical instruments including syringes, needles, scalpel, scissors, forceps, suture needles, sterile drapes, towels, razor, cotton etc.

LUBRICATION AND DYSTOCIA
• Common lubricants are linseed oil, liquid paraffin, jellies, mineral oil etc.
• In difficult or prolonged dystocia, use of lubricants is essential.
• Epidural anaesthesia is necessary, when much lubrication is required because it (epidural anaesthesia) prevents straining and throwing out of lubricant.
• Epidural anaesthesia also cause sufficient relaxation so that the lubricant can flow about and cover the foetus, uterine wall, cervical wall and vaginal walls.
• Lubricants should be rubbed on the foetus and wall of the birth-canal.
• In case of prolonged operations, the lubricant should be applied two or more times or as frequently as the foetus or birth-canal becomes dry.

EXERCISE :

1. Observe different types of obstetrical instruments carefully and practice their use on dummy foetus in phantom box.

2. What is use of rope and snare ?
Ans.

3. Write the name of hooks which are used for traction of live foetus.
Ans.

4. Write the name of hooks which are used for traction of dead foetus.
Ans.

5. What are the sites of application of Harris hook and Obermayer's hook ?
Ans.

6. Which hook is the most commonly used during traction of foetus in breech presentation ?
Ans.

7. Sharp hooks should be covered by a cork at the pointed end at the time of carrying inside the genital tract. Why ?

Ans.

8. What is the difference between sharp hooks and blunt hooks?

Ans.

9. What is the difference between short hooks and long hooks?

Ans.

10. What is use of chisel ?

Ans.

11. What is the use of spatula ?

Ans.

12. How does Cammerer's torsion fork help in rotation of foetus ? Explain.

Ans.

13. How does Kuhn's crutch help in repelling the foetus inside the uterus ? Describe in detail.

Ans.

14. What is the total length of Thygesen's foetotome ?

Ans.

15. Why the short hooks have an eye at one end ?

Ans.

✺ ✺ ✺ ✺ ✺

Cowards die many times before their death; the valiants never taste of death but once.

Chapter 23

An Approach to a Case of Dystocia

Cases of dystocia should be attended without any delay. The history of case should be taken and a general clinical assessment and examination should be carried out.

Assistance required :

- Ideally the obstetrician should have the help of **three assistants.** One to manage the head of the patient and two to assist with foetal delivery at her rear end and to prevent the cow from swinging her rear end around during examination and treatment.

Restraint of the patient :

- The head should be tied low to allow the cow to lie down with ease during delivery, if she wishes.

Sedation :

- In some cases, especially with nervous unhandled heifers, sedation with xylazine may be required before internal examination for safety.
- Sufficient sedation is normally achieved by giving the patient 5 mg. of xylazine per 100 kg. body weight by intramuscular injection.
- **Xylazine may** increase the strength of myometrial contractions **but this normally does not cause any problem.**
- Heavy sedation should be avoided.

Uterine relaxation :

- This may occasionally be required if strong myometrial contraction are obstructing an obstetrical manoeuvre such as correction of malposture.
- **Clenbuterol at a dose of 300 mg** for the average cow, given by

intramuscular injection will cause uterine relaxation and also **reduce the strength of uterine contractions due to use of xylazine.**

Epidural anaesthesia :

- This is only required at calving if intense maternal straining makes procedures such as foetal repulsion very difficult.
- Frequent defaecation is suppressed but myometrial activity is unaffected.
- In the average cow, 5-7 ml. of 2% lignocaine should be given which is effective in controlling straining as well as maintaining the patient's ability to stand.

Equipment :

- Water-proof parturition gown and gumboots.
- Unless infection is suspected or the obstetrician's arms are sensitive to bovine vaginal secretions, protective sleeves and gloves are not normally worn.
- **Three nylon calving ropes** of different colours with short wooden cylindrical handles.
- A sterile surgical kit for caesarean section.
- A foetotomy set.
- Lubricant – **Synthetic colloidal gels** are very useful and at **least 750 ml should be available for calving**. Soap and water are the traditional obstetrical lubricant but it tends to disperse natural lubricants. Liquid paraffin may also be used as lubricant.
- Drugs : Oxytocin, calcium borogluconate, dextrose solutions, injectable antibiotics, uterine pessaries, tetanus anti-toxin, clenbuterol or **isoxsuprine.**
- Warm water – 5 litres.
- Equipment for resuscitation of the calf should be ready. Particularly **doxapram hydrochloride** should be always loaded in a syringe.

General clinical examination of cow :

- Special attention must be paid to the cow's udder to ensure that there is no evidence of **developing coliform mastitis.**
- Foetal movement should be noticed at the cow's left flank and if this is vigorous, it indicates the placental separation which causes foetal anoxia and hypermotility.

133

- Signs of placental separation may be seen at the vulva if part of the chorioallantois with detached cotyledons are visible (see Fig 23.1).

- A light yellowish green vaginal discharge may indicate foetal anoxia with associated **expulsion of meconium.**

Vaginal examination :

- The lubricated hand should be inserted into the vagina and the condition of cervix is assessed. If the **cervix is closed, the protruded but soft external os can be identified but fully dilated cervix cannot be distinguished because the vaginal walls remain continued with the uterine wall.**

- It is quite easy to fail to recognize the closed cervix in cases where the foetal fore limbs have entered in the pelvic canal. The limb may appear within the vagina but still enclosed in the foetal membranes. In fact, the closed cervix is ventrally displaced and the **calf is still fully within the uterus** (see Fig. 23.2). The error can be minimized by careful and systemic examination of the anterior vagina.

- The size of pelvis should also be determined whether it is narrow or normal (see Fig. 23.3).

- After rupture of amnion, the foetus is examined with the hand to determine its presentation, position and posture.

- Ascertain whether the fore limbs or hind limbs are present in birth-canal (see Fig. 23.4).

- The interesting techniques of vaginal examination in the bitch and sow are described in Fig. 23.5, 23.6, 23.7, and 23.8.

CLINICAL POINTERS
- If the obstetrician's hand can be passed with ease around the foetal shoulders within maternal pelvis then foetal delivery *per vaginum* is normally possible (see Fig. 23.3) in anterior presentation.
- In posterior presentation if the hand can pass readily between the maternal pelvis and the hind quarters of the calf including the thighs, hips and tail then vaginal delivery is likely to be possible in posterior presentation.
- It must be remembered that viability of the calf is often higher after caesarean section than after forced extraction.

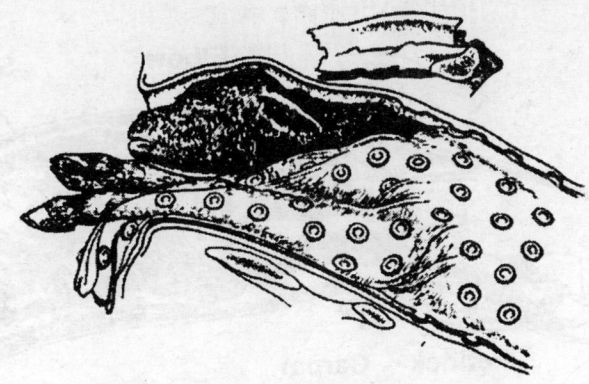

Fig. 23.1 : Sign of placental separation

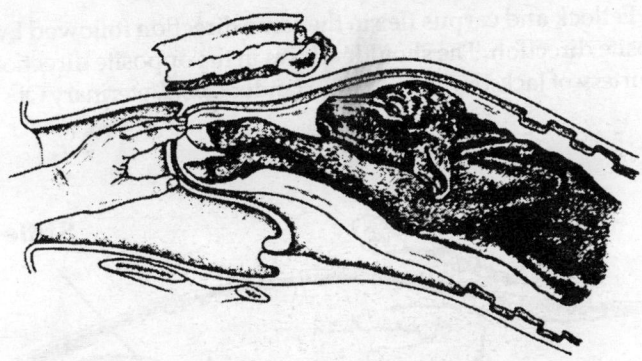

Fig. 23.2 : Failure to recognise the closed cervixs.

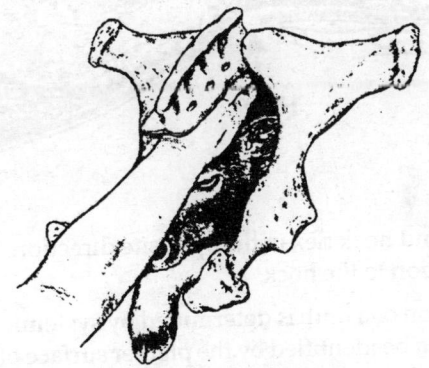

Fig. 23.3 : Comparison of the size of the foetus and birth canal. This examination is normally carried out as part of the vaginal examination. The lubricated hand is passed over the presenting parts of the foetus within the pelvis and is then moved in a circular fashion around the foetus, estimating the amount space between foetus and pelvis.

135

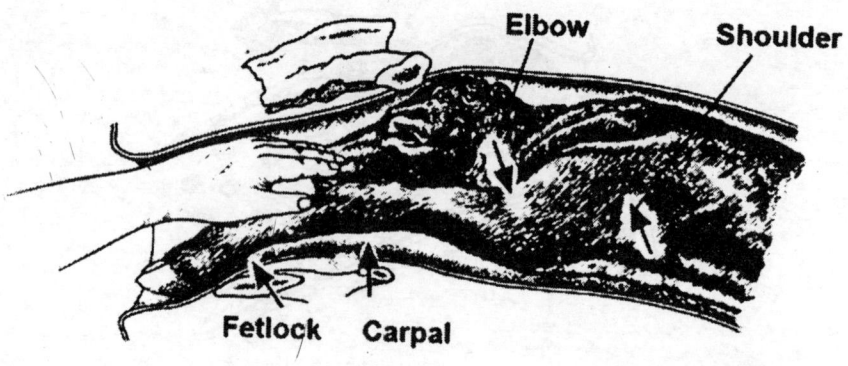

Fore limb : Fetlock and carpus flex in the same direction followed by elbow in the opposite direction. The shoulder flexes in the opposite direction to the elbow. (Courtesy of Jackson, P.G.G. 1995. Handbook of Veterinary Obstetrics).

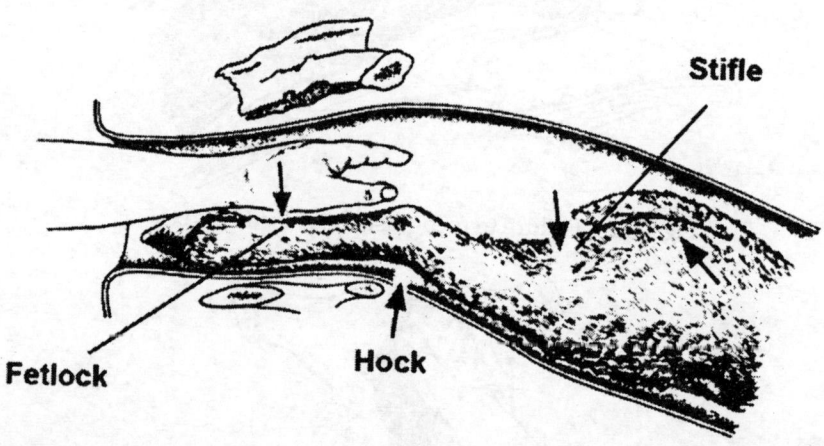

Hind limb : Fetlock and hock flex in the opposite direction. The stifle flexes in the opposite direction to the hock.

Fig. 23.4 : Identification of a limb is determined by systemic palpation of its joint. The fore limb can be identified by the planter surface of the hoof facing downwards whereas in case of hind limbs, the planter surface of the hof faces upwards. Proof is obtained by noting the direction of flexion of the limb joints. (Courtesy of Jackson, P.G.G. 1995. Handbook of Veterinary Obstetrics).

An interesting technique of vaginal examination of a bitch just before parturition

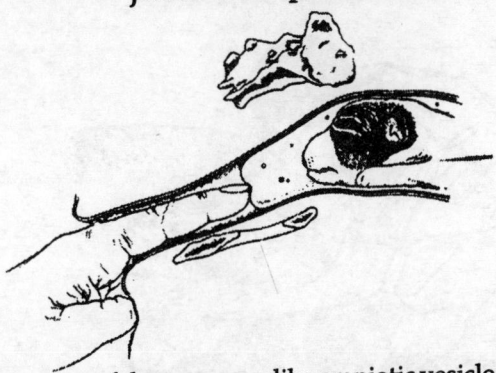

Fig. 23.5 : Palpation of the gossamer like amniotic vesicle which may indicate the approach of a foetus.The presence of an approaching amniotic vesicle normally means that a foetus is also approaching. Palpation of a few minutes later will often reveal the foetal head (see next figures). (Courtesy of Jackson, P.G.G. 1995. Handbook of Veterinary Obstetrics).

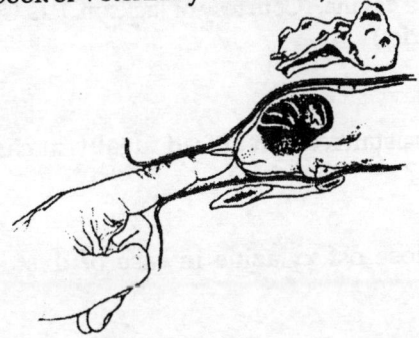

Fig. 23.6 : The foetal head may be palpable shortly after the amniotic vescile. (Courtesy of Jackson, P.G.G. 1995. Handbook of Veterinary Obstetrics).

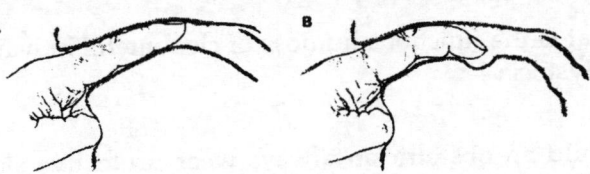

Fig. 23.7 : Assessing the tone of the anterior vagina. In the average bitch, the cervix and uterus cannot be palpated *per vaginum* but the palpable characteristics of anterior vagina give some indication of what is happening at the cervix and within the uterus. For example A. Pronounced tone indicate satisfactory muscular activity in the uterus, B. Flaccidity indicates uterine inertia. (Courtesy of Jackson, P.G.G. 1995. Handbook of Veterinary Obstetrics).

An interesting technique of vaginal examination of a sow just before parturition

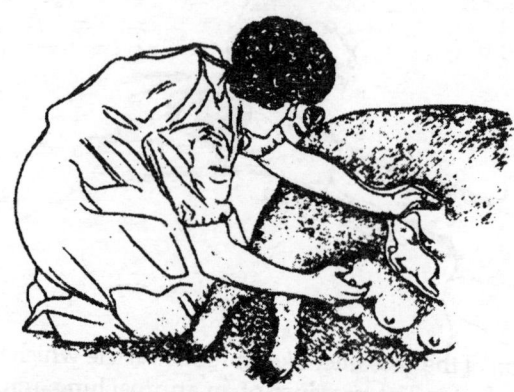

Fig. 23.8 : It is usually more convenient to encourage the sow to remain in the lateral recumbency during vaginal examination. Gentle massage of udder encourage most sows to remain in lateral recumbency even when the hand is introduced into the vagina. (Courtesy of Jackson, P.G.G. 1995. Handbook of Veterinary Obstetrics).

EXERCISE :

1.   How many assistants are required ideally in case of dystocia in large animals ?

Ans.

2.   What is the dose osf xylazine in case of dystocia in cattle for sedation ?

Ans.

3.   Does xylazine increase the strength of myometrial contraction ?

Ans.

4.   What is the function and dose of clenbuterol in handling a case of dystocia ?

Ans.

5.   Should an obstetrician always wear protective sleeve during correction of dystocia ?

Ans.

6.   Write the name of different lubricants used during correction of dystocia.

Ans.

7. How much volume of lubricane is required per calving ?

Ans.

8. What will be your interpretation when a cow is having a light yellowish green discharge during dystocia ?

Ans.

9. Write the disadvantages of premature rupture of water bag.

Ans.

❋ ❋ ❋ ❋ ❋

Discussion is an exchange of knowledge but argument is an exchange of ignorance.

139

Chapter 24

Evidence of Foetal Life

It is important to evaluate vital signs of the unborn calf because they influence the choice of the obstetric treatment.

SIGNS OF LIFE OF A FOETUS :

Anterior presentation :

Signs of life of a foetus in anterior presentation can be determined by the interdigital claw reflex, swallowing reflex, palpebral reflex, palpation of heart beat and pulsation in the umbilical cord.

Interdigital claw reflex :
- It is stimulated by firmly pinching the inter digital web. Positive response to pedal withdrawal is the sign of life of a foetus.
- A vigorous (normal and live) foetus usually withdraws its foot only once.
- When the reaction is exaggerated or in the form of pedaling motions, it may indicate **hypoxia and/ or acidosis.**
- When the head has entered the pelvic canal, the interdigital claw reflex is sometimes absent even though the foetus is normal.
- During straining, it may give false indication due to straining pressure; limbs of foetus remain pressed in the birth canal but when pressure relaxes, it (limb) seems to retract both in live and dead foetus.

Swallowing reflex :
- It is stimulated by applying **pressure on the base of the tongue.**
- A **vigorous calf** will usually react by swallowing or by making gentle sucking motions.
- **Exaggerated** sucking reflex indicates **hypoxia and/ or serious acidosis.**

Palpebral reflex :
- It is stimulated by placing slight **pressure on the eyeballs,** the eye reflex can be felt as a vibration of the eyes or as a movement of the eyelids.

CLINICAL POINTERS
• With worsening condition, these reflexes disappear in definite order. The interdigital claw reflex is negative first, and the eye reflex remains positive for the longest period.
• A positive response indicates a calf is still alive; however, a negative response does not always mean that it is dead.

DO YOU KNOW?
During hypoxia, blood circulation is directed towards the heart and the brain, which allow oxygen supply to the heart and the brain as long as possible at the expenses of peripheral tissues, particularly the muscles. Therefore anaerobic glycolysis and accumulation of lactic acid occurs first in muscles and decreases their reactivity. This explains why reflexes of the extremities become negative first.

Palpation of heart beat :

- The heart beat is palpated by passing the hand between the front legs of the foetus and by grasping the sternum from below, preferably with fingers on the left side of the chest wall.
- The normal heart rate should be about **120 beats/ minute.**
- The drop in heart beats indicates that the foetus is in poor condition.

Pulsation in umbilical cord :

- The umbilical cord can be located by searching the area between the curvature of the last ribs and the flaccid abdomen.
- Pulsation and tension of the vessels can be best evaluated by slight pressure on the umbilical cord.
- During normal parturition, pulse frequency gradually increases from **about 90 to 120/ minute.**
- Drop in pulse frequency indicates that the calf is in poor condition.

Posterior presentation :

Vitality of a foetus in posterior presentation can be determined by the pedal reflex, anal reflex and pulsation in the umbilical cord.

Anal reflex :

- It is stimulated as a constriction of the anal sphincter when a finger is pushed against or into the anus.

- This reflex is **not very reliable** because it is absent in some vigorous foetus.

Interdigital claw reflex :

- The interdigital claw reflex of the rear feet is lost sooner than that of the front feet and can sometimes be negative in a live foetus.
- The pedal reflex can be absent when a **live foetus is wedged in the birth canal.**
- Therefore its prognostic value is not as good as when performed on the front feet.

Pulsation of the umbilical cord :

- The umbilical cord can **always be easily reached in calves in posterior presentation and its evaluation is always effective** in determining vitality of the calf.

Other evidences of foetal life :

Inspection of mucus membrane :

- If the foetal head is protruding from the vulva, the ocular mucus membrane may be inspected.
- The mucus membranes should be **pink in a healthy well-oxygenated calf. Cynosis** indicates low degree of hypoxia. Extreme **pallor** mucus membranes suggest that the foetus is severely anoxic.

Evidence of foetal death :

- Absence of positive signs of life as mentioned above.
- After 12 hours of the foetal death, **blood staining of the amniotic fluid** occurs.
- After 72 hours of the foetal death, development of **corneal opacity** commences.
- Degeneration and separation of the placenta with loss of foetal fluid.

OBSERVATIONS:

Date ....

- Case No. ....
- Species ....

- Age ....
- Parity ....
- Presentation/ Position/ Posture ....
- Interdigital claw reflex ....
- Swallowing reflex ....
- Palpebral reflex ....
- Heart beat ..../min.
- Pulse (umbilical cord) rate ..../min.
- Anal reflex ....
- Ocular mucus membrane ....
- Prognosis ....
- Obstetrical operation used ....·.....
- · Result ....

EXERCISE :

1. Write the order of disappearing of reflexes in a poor condition of foetus.

Ans.

2. How will you locate the umbilical cord in anterior presentation?

Ans.

3. In which presentation, location of umbilical cord is easier ?

Ans.

4. Which method is reliable to see the evidence of life of a foetus in a posterior presentation ?

Ans.

5. When does the pedal reflex remain absent in posterior presentation ?

Ans.

❈ ❈ ❈ ❈ ❈

There is always a way to acquire knowledge, always a way to get ahead if the will to learn is there.
— *J.C. Roberts*

Chapter 25

Vaginal Delivery by Using Mutation and Force Traction

Mutation : *It is defined as those operations by which a foetus is returned to a normal presentation, position and posture by repulsion, rotation, version and adjustment of flexed extremity.*

Repulsion or retropulsion :

This consists of pushing the foetus forward into the uterus from the birth canal to make adequate space for the correction of position and posture.

- This is done either with operator's arm or with the help of some instruments like **Kuhn's crutch repeller**. The crutch or hand is placed over the **chest** beneath the neck of the foetus in **anterior presentation** or **above the ischial arch** in the perineal region in **posterior presentation.**

- Before doing the actual operation, liquid paraffin or linseed oil should be used to lubricate the uterine wall.

- If water bag has already been ruptured, Kuhn's crutch should be applied.

- Repulsion is very effective in standing position of dam.

- However, the use of such instrument increases uterine contractions and any slip from the slippery surface of the foetus leading to severe injuries to the uterus. Therefore, the instrument should be used very carefully.

Rotation :

"It is the turning of foetus on its long axis to bring the foetus into dorso-sacral position (anterior presentation) or lumbo-sacral position (posterior presentation).

- Malposition is corrected by rotation of foetal body after retropulsion.

- Epidural anaesthesia and adequate lubrication of birth canal facilitates easy repulsion and rotation.
- If fore limbs or hind limbs are seen in the birth-canal, secure them and pass hand between the body of foetus and the uterus and try to rotate the foetus into desired direction.
- Different detorsion rods can be used for this purpose like **Cammerer's torsion fork** (Fig. 25.1 & 25.2).

Version:

"It is rotation of foetus on its transverse axis into an anterior or posterior presentation."

OR

"Rotate the foetus on its transverse axis by repelling one end and applying traction on the other end to bring it into either anterior longitudinal or posterior longitudinal presentation" (see Fig. 25.3a & 25.3b).

- It is done by long handle eye hook or hand alone or Kuhn's crutch.
- Version includes two important movements- **repulsion** and **evolution.** After repelling the foetus into the uterus, the posterior limbs are seized, corded and pulled towards the pelvis and simultaneously, the anterior parts are being repelled towards the cranial end. This is evolution.

Extension and adjustment of the extremities:

"The correction of abnormal posture of head, neck and limbs of the foetus is called extension or adjustment of the extremities" (see Fig. 25.10-25.20).

Force traction / extraction:

"The withdrawal of foetus from birth canal of the dam by application of force is called force traction".

- Such a force may be developed by cords, hooks and forceps.
- Lubrication of the genitalia is essential for forced traction.
- Traction should be simultaneous, without jerk and should be applied during expulsive efforts of the dam.

Application of ropes in force traction :

- If ropes are to be placed on both the head and legs of the calf, **the head rope should always be placed first** because if the legs ropes are attached first, there may be insufficient room or space for the head rope to be placed in position with ease.

- **Application of head-rope :** A large loop is made as the end of a rope. The loop is carried into the vagina and placed carefully behind both ears of the calf (see Fig. 25.4 a & 4b). The lower end of loop is placed within the mouth of the calf before it is tightened (see Fig. 25.4c). *The head rope should never be looped around the lower jaw because traction may cause serious damage to the jaw.*

- **Application of the leg-ropes :** A loop is made at the end of the calving rope. The loop is slipped over calf's foot. The loop is held in position with one hand and is then pulled tight with other hand (see Fig. 25.4d, 4e & 4f). *Great care must be taken to ensure that the leg-ropes are secured above the fetlock; if they are applied below the fetlock, damage to the joint or the hooves may occur.*

Direction of pull:

- As the calf enters the pelvic inlet the pull should be **directed dorsally backwards.** As the head passes through the pelvis, it should be **directed horizontally backwards** and once the head has passed through the pelvis the direction of pull should be **downwards torwards the cow's hock.** The subtle (artful) alteration of the direction of pull will allow advantage of the greatest diameter of the pelvis and also allow the calf to maintain a profile that will reduce its diameter.

- During delivery, **one forelegs should be pulled slightly in advance of the other. This reduces the width of the foetal shoulder as it passes through the pelvis** (see Fig. 25.6).

  Pulling should be timed to coincide with straining of the cow. When pulling commences, traction is applied to each rope in turn right leg, left leg and head (see Fig. 25.6).

- Once the head and shoulders have passed through the vulva, **traction should be applied simultaneously to the head and legs.**

- Once the head and shoulders have passed through the vulva, **umbilical cord gets compressed. Therefore at this stage, delivery should be completed as soon as possible, because foetus can only survive for about 3-6 minutes without access to fresh** supply of oxygen.

Principles of force traction :

- **Cross traction** : Cross traction of fore limbs in anterior presentation helps to *reduce the shoulder dimension of the foetus* and helps in smooth passage of the thorax.

- **Alternate traction** : Simultaneous traction on the head and limbs has resulted in direct entry of the widest diameter of the fore part of the body into the pelvis which consequently interferes with delivery (see Fig. 25.7 & 25.8). Therefore, alternate traction of limbs results in unequal entry of the shoulder and elbow joint into the pelvic cavity, which *results in oblique passage of the shoulder girdle through the pelvis* (see Fig. 25.6 & 25.9).

IMPORTANT POINTS
• Whenever calving aids or pulleys are used, the obstetrician must always be aware of the potential force of their pull. The pulleys or aids can exert a pulling force of 400 kg *compared with a force of 200 kg exterted by two persons pulling and the normal expulsive force of the calving cow is estimated to be 75 kg.*
• The amount of force to be applied depends on species and condition causing dystocia. However, in general, *it should not exceed four men power in large animals.*
• *Pulling should never be started with the calf in posterior presentation unless the obstetrician is sure that sufficient help is available.*
Reason : Delivery of the calf in posterior presentation is more hazardous than the calf in anterior presentation; because the umbilical cord breaks early in the delivery in comparison to anterior presentation. Therefore delivery should be completed as soon as possible after starting the force traction otherwise calf may become anoxic and inhale amniotic fluid and drown.

CLINICAL POINTERS
• If the foetus fails to move at all during attempted delivery traction, it should be stopped and the foetus is re-examined to ensure that the posture of calf is as expected.
• If no progress is made within 10 minutes traction; it should be stopped and the calf should be delivered by caesarean section or by foetotomy.

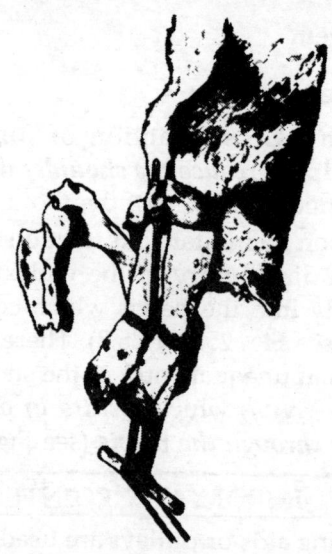

Fig. 25. 1 : See the method of rotation of the foetus in anterior presentation, from the ventral to the dorsal position using the torsion fork. (Courtesy of Benesch, F. and Wright, J.G. 2001. Veterinary Obstetrics. Greenworld Publishers).

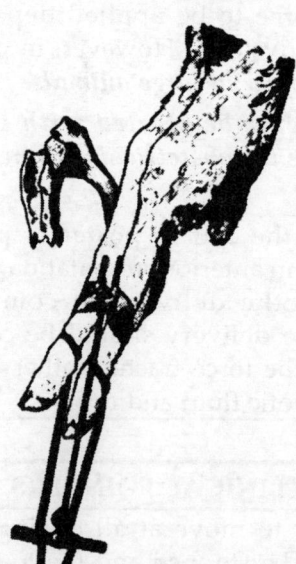

Fig. 25. 2 : See the use of the torsion fork for rotating the foetus from the ventral position in posterior presentation and extended posture. (Courtesy of Benesch, F. and Wright, J.G. 2001. Veterinary Obstetrics. Greenworld Publishers).

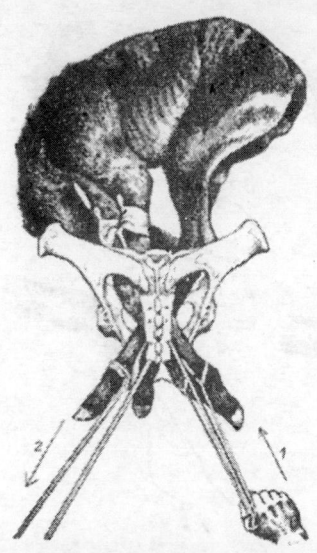

Fig. 25.3a : Ventro-transverse presentation with ventral displacement of the head. Turning of the foetus by the crutch-cuff method is commenced. Pressure against the fore part of the body, and simultaneous light traction on the hind limbs (first stage). (Courtesy of Benesch, F. and Wright, J.G. 2001. Veterinary Obstetrics. Greenworld Publishers).

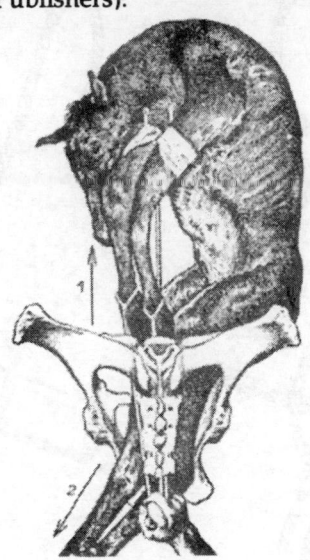

Fig. 25.3b : Turning of the foetus from ventro-transverse to posterior presentation, lateral position, completed (second stage). The foetus is extracted after removal of the crutch. (Courtesy of Benesch, F. and Wright, J.G. 2001. Veterinary Obstetrics. Greenworld Publishers).

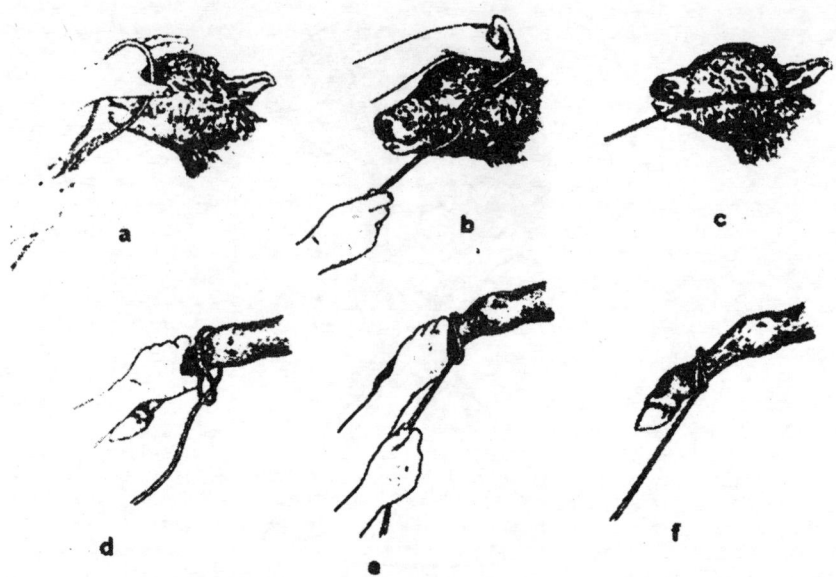

Fig. 25.4 : Methods of application of calving ropes. (Courtesy of Jackson, P.G.G. 1995. Handbook of Veterinary Obstetrics. W.B. Saunders Company Limited).

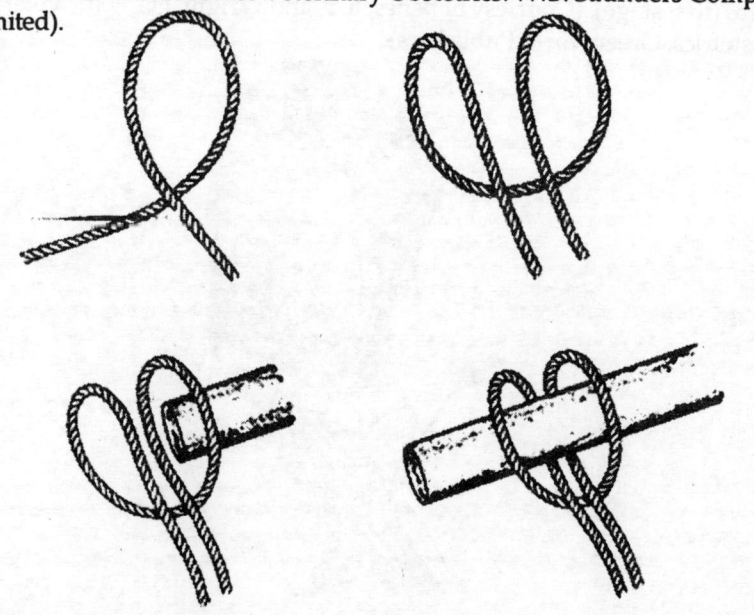

Fig. 25.5 : Method of application of rope over wooden handle. (Courtesy of Jackson, P.G.G. 1995. Handbook of Veterinary Obstetrics. W.B. Saunders Company Limited)

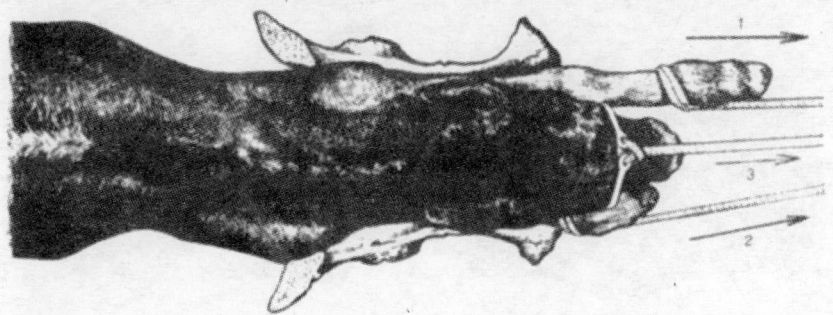

Fig. 25. 6 : Force traction on one fore limb has resulted in unequal entry of the shoulder and elbow joints into the pelvic inlet and consequently, oblique passage of the shoulder through the pelvis (**correct method**). Fore traction should be applied to each rope in turn, left leg (1), right leg (2) and head (3). (Courtesy of Benesch, F. and Wright, J.G. 2001. Veterinary Obstetrics. Greenworld Publishers).

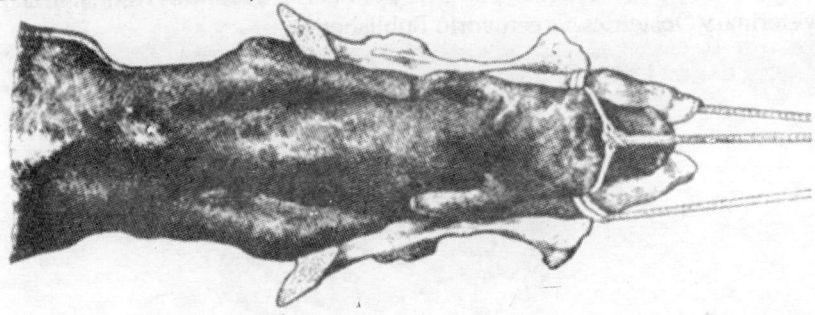

Fig. 25. 7 : Simultaneous traction on the head and limbs has resulted in directed entry of the widest diameter of the fore part of the body into the pelvis and consequently interference with delivery (**incorrect method**). (Courtesy of Benesch, F. and Wright, J.G. 2001. Veterinary Obstetrics. Greenworld Publishers).

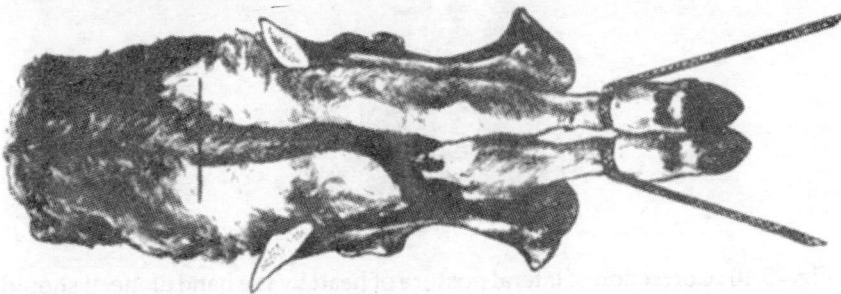

Fig. 25. 8 : Simultaneous traction applied to both extremities has resulted in obstruction because direct entry of the largest diameter of the foetal pelvis into the maternal pelvis (**incorrect method**). (Courtesy of Benesch, F. and Wright, J.G. 2001. Veterinary Obstetrics. Greenworld Publishers).

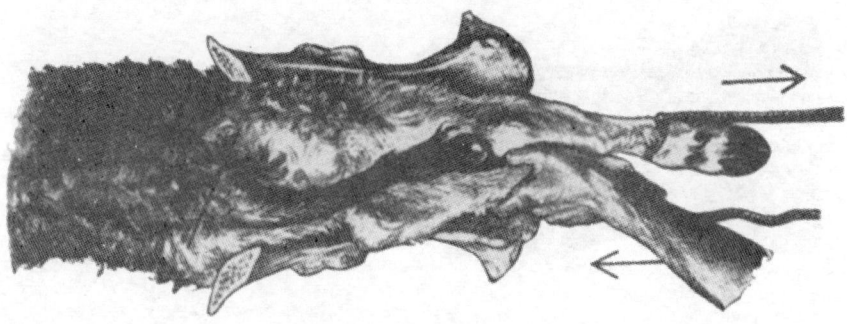

Fig. 25.9 : Unilateral traction (the opposite limb being repelled as far as possible in the genital passage) causes an oblique position of the foetal pelvis and therefore an easier entry into the maternal pelvis. After one extremity has been drawn back sufficiently, simultaneous traction is exerted on the two limbs (**correct method**). (Courtesy of Benesch, F. and Wright, J.G. 2001. Veterinary Obstetrics. Greenworld Publishers).

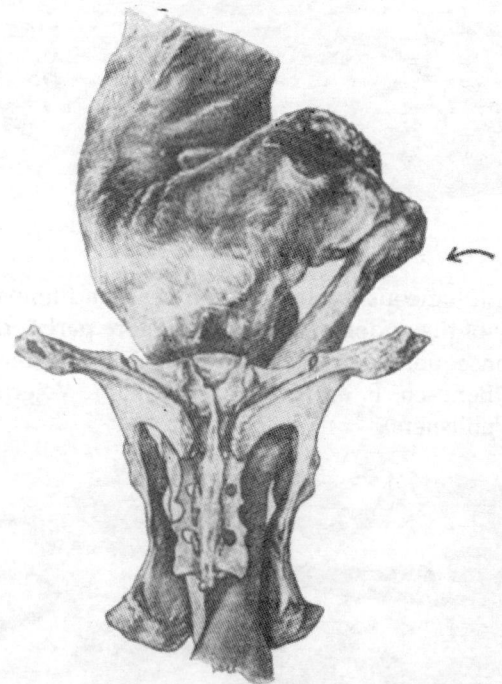

Fig. 25.10 : Correction of lateral posture of head by the hand alone. It should always be remembered that cup-shaped hand should apply over the mouth of the foetus which protects the uterine wall against the sharp teeth as well as act as a guide. (Courtesy of Benesch, F. and Wright, J.G. 2001. Veterinary Obstetrics. Greenworld Publishers).

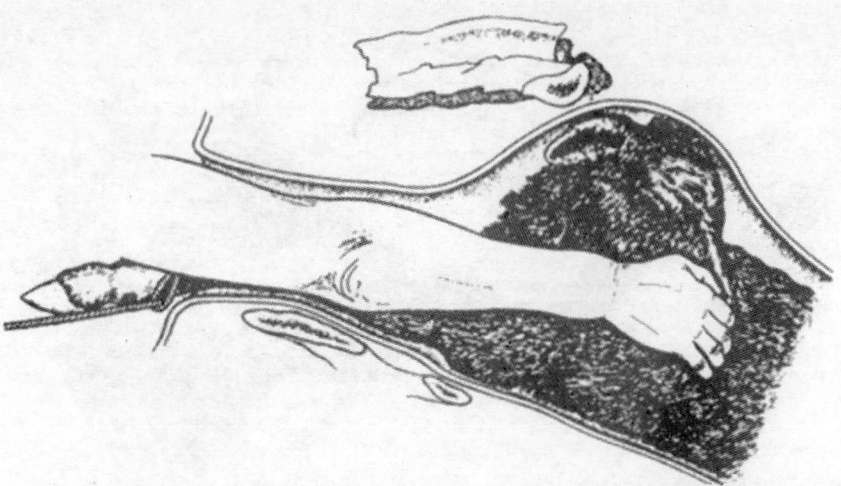

Fig. 25.11 : Correction of foetal malposture - lateral deviation of the head. The muzzle is located and covered by the obstertrician's hand before being guided round the arc of a circle and upto the pelvis. (Courtesy of Jackson, P.G.G. 1995. Handbook of Veterinary Obstetrics. W.B. Saunders Company Limited).

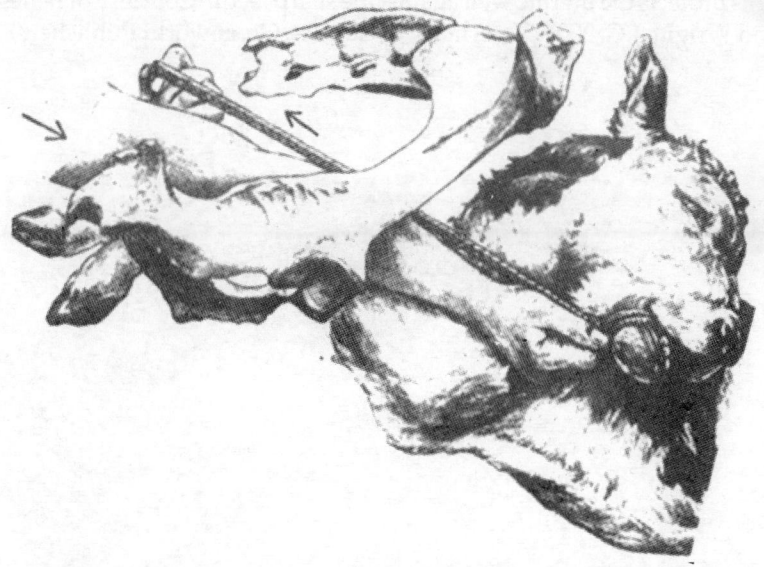

Fig. 25.12 : Correction of lateral deviation of head with mandibular snare or rope (stage I). It should always be remembered that mandibular snare must not be used for traction because it causes serious damage to the jaw. The mandibular snare should be used only for redirection of the displaced head. (Courtesy of Benesch, F. and Wright, J.G. 2001. Veterinary Obstetrics. Greenworld Publishers).

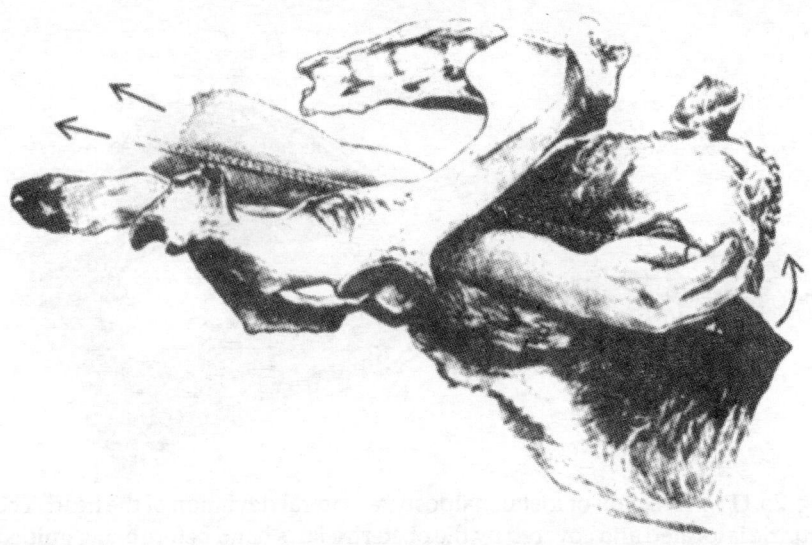

Fig. 25.13 : Correction of lateral deviation of head with mandibular snare (stage II). See the placement of hand over the mouth which acts as a guide as well as protects the uterine wall against the sharp teeth. (Courtesy of Benesch, F. and Wright, J.G. 2001. Veterinary Obstetrics. Greenworld Publishers).

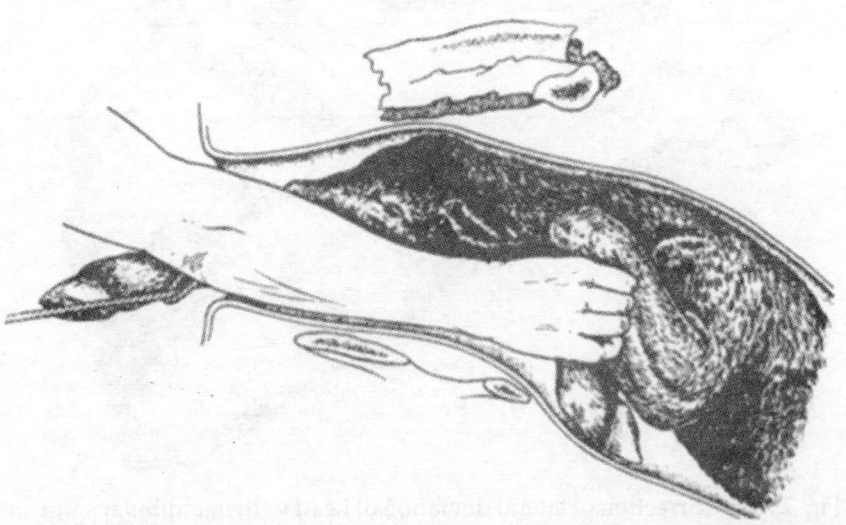

Fig. 25.14 : Correction of foetal malposture-carpal flexion (stage-I). Raise the flexed carpus against the side of the foetal neck by grasping the meta-carpus. (Courtesy of Jackson, P.G.G. 1995. Handbook of Veterinary Obstetrics. W.B. Saunders Company Limited).

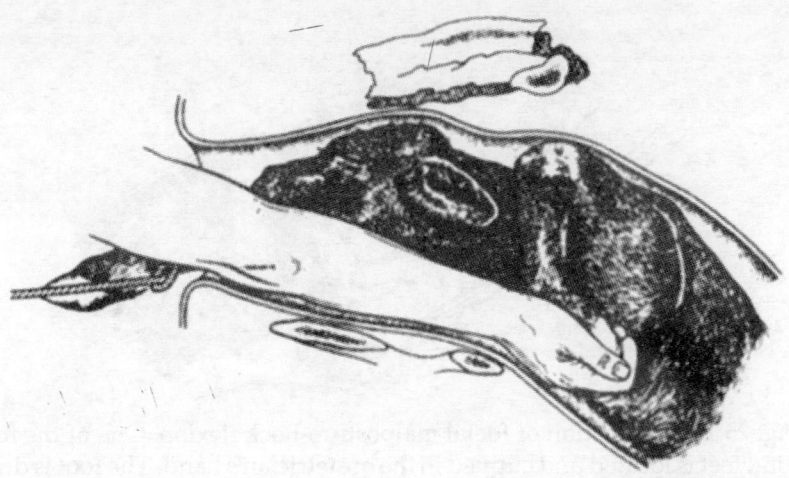

Fig. 25.15 : Correction of foetal malposture-carpal flexion (stage II). Once the foot is within reach, it must be cupped in the hand and brought carefully into the pelvis. It should always be kept in mind during correction of any type of retention of fore limb, the foetal foot should always be brought in the pelvis in the cupped hand because it prevents injury to the birth canal by the foot. (Courtesy of Jackson, P.G.G. 1995. Handbook of Veterinary Obstetrics. W.B. Saunders Company Limited).

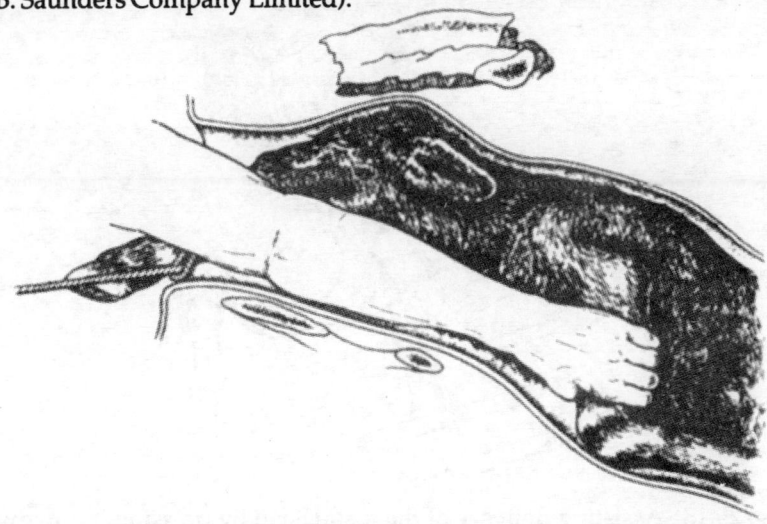

Fig. 25.16 : Correction of foetal malposture-shoulder flexion. The limb should be grasped and brought up into the carpal flexion position and then the foot is brought into the pelvis as described in previous figures. In some cases, ropes are used for traction. (Courtesy of Jackson, P.G.G. 1995. Handbook of Veterinary Obstetrics. W.B. Saunders Company Limited).

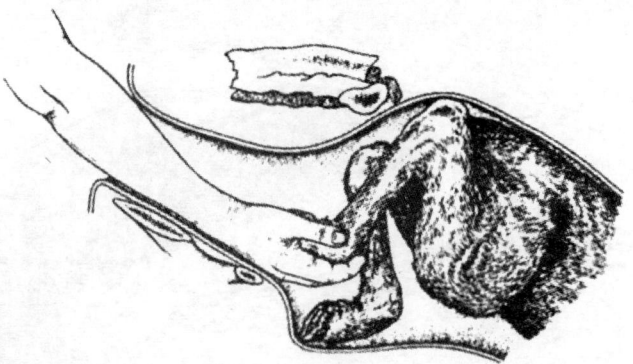

Fig. 25.17 : Correction of foetal malposture-hock flexion. One of the foetal hind feet is located and cupped in the obstetrician's hand. The foot is drawn backward and upward in the arc of a circle into the pelvis. (Courtesy of Jackson, P.G.G. 1995. Handbook of Veterinary Obstetrics. W.B. Saunders Company Limited).

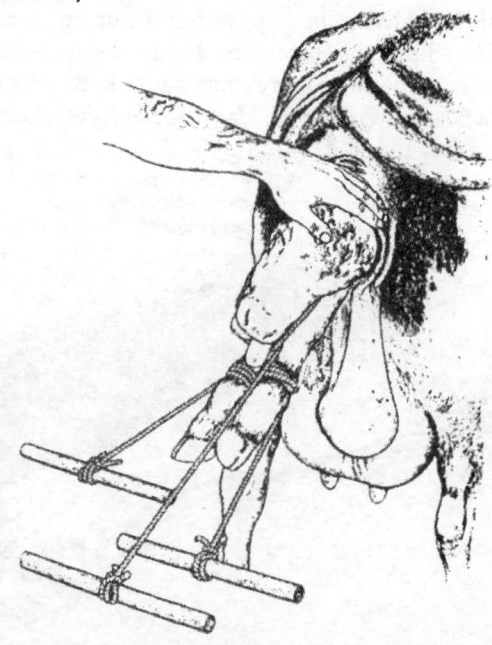

Fig. 25.18 : Assisting delivery of the foetal head by pressing it downwards and elevating the dorsal vaginal wall because the dorsal vaginal wall is quite fragile at this point and the poll of the foetal head can easily stretch and rupture the tissues, allowing prolapse of sub mucosal fat to occur. Therefore, damage can be prevented by doing this. (Courtesy of Jackson, P.G.G. 1995. Handbook of Veterinary Obstetrics. W.B. Saunders Company Limited).

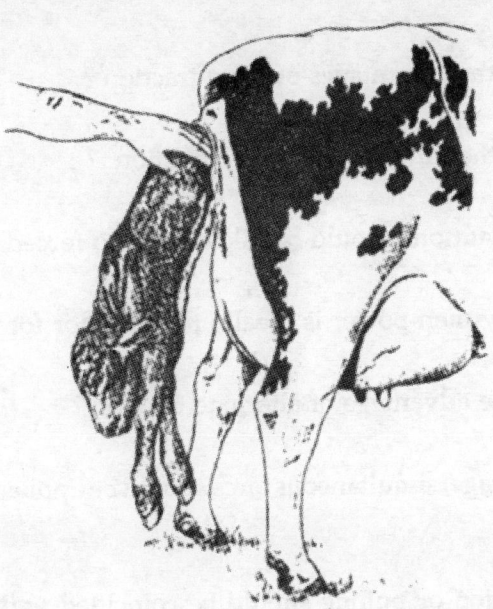

Fig. 25.19 : Stifle lock can arrest the foetus during delivery. (Courtesy of Jackson, P.G.G. 1995. Handbook of Veterinary Obstetrics. W.B. Saunders Company Limited).

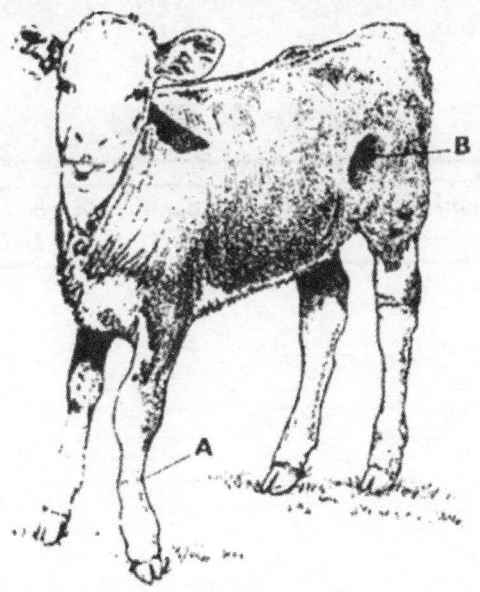

Fig. 25.20 : Calf showing injuries caused by excessive traction A. Fractured metacarpus B. Quadriceps atrophy by femoral nerve paralysis. (Courtesy of Jackson, P.G.G. 1995. Handbook of Veterinary Obstetrics. W.B. Saunders Company Limited).

157

EXERCISE :

1. What are the advantages of force traction ?

Ans.

2. What are the limitations of force traction ?

Ans.

3. What precautions should be taken prior to forced extraction ?

Ans.

4. How many men-power is ideally required for force traction ?

Ans.

5. What is the advantage of alternate traction ?

Ans.

6. In which stage, simultaneous force should be applied during force traction ?

Ans.

7. Force traction or pulling should be coincided with straining of cow. Why ?

Ans.

8. Practice mutations and forced traction, by using dummy calf in phantom box.

❊ ❊ ❊ ❊ ❊

Half the ills of mankind are due to ignorance, the other half arise from egotism.
– Lala Har Dayal ·

Chapter 26

Techniques of Foetotomy

Foetotomy (embryotomy) :

Removal or division of certain parts of foetus to reduce the size of the foetus is called foetotomy.

- Foetotomy is used most commonly in cattle, occasionally in horses, rarely in sheep and goats and almost never in pigs and small animals.
- **Complete foetotomy :** *When a whole foetus is divided into small pieces, the operation is known as complete foetotomy.*
- **Incomplete foetotomy :** *When a small part of the foetus is removed, the operation is known as incomplete foetotomy.*
- Two techniques of foetotomy are in practice : **subcutaneous** and **percutaneous.**

Subcutaneous foetotomy : *Removal of decorticated limb (skinless limb) to reduce the size of foetus is called subcutaneous foetotomy.*

Technique of subcutaneous foetotomy :

Fore limb :
- The fore limb is snared around the **pastern instead of around the fetlock** (generally, during traction, fetlock is used for application of rope).
- Continuous traction is applied on the snare by one assistant
- A small incision is made with a scalpel into the skin in front of fetlock joint.
- A longitudinal incision is made with the help of Robert's foetotomy knife from the fetlock to the scapula (see Fig. 26.1).
- Dissect the skin (separation of skin from the muscles) with the help of fingers around the leg and extend it to the scapular region.
- This is followed by division of the muscles connecting the scapula and thorax by Robert's knife.
- Next step is to **disarticulate the fetlock joint without severing the skin** (see Fig. 26.2).

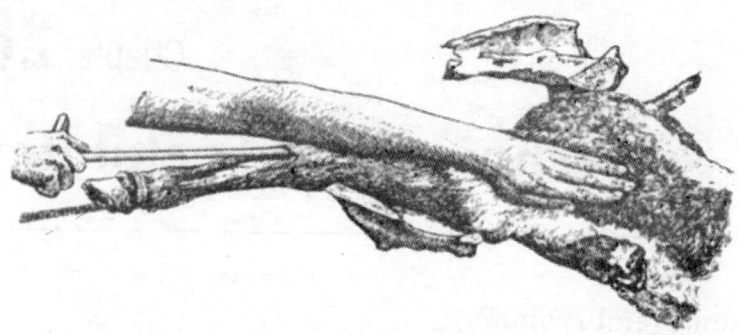

Fig. 26.1 : Subcutaneous removal of the extended fore limb (Stage I). The other fore limb has been flexed and replaced in the uterus to provide more space. The skin is being incised or separated from fetlock to the scapula, using Robert's foetotomy knife or Keller's spatula. (Courtesy of Benesch, F. and Wright, J.G. 2001. Veterinary Obstetrics. Greenworld Publishers).

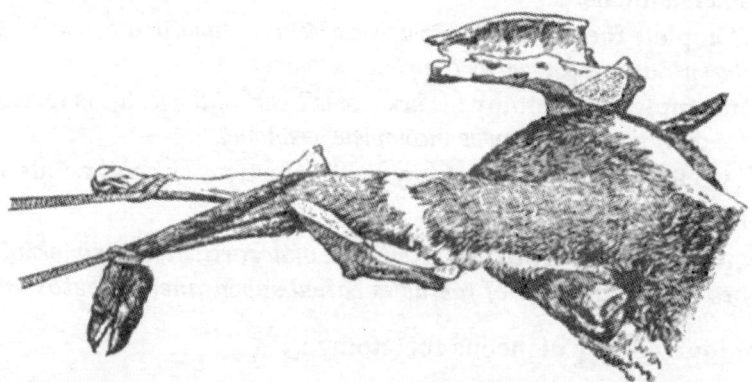

Fig. 26.2 : Subcutaneous removal of the extended fore limb (Stage II). After disarticulation of the fetlock joint, the limb is removed "through the skin" and traction is applied to the denuded limb. Note that the preservation of the digits with the skin serves for effective attachment of the traction cord. (Courtesy of Benesch, F. and Wright, J.G. 2001. Veterinary Obstetrics. Greenworld Publishers).

- Now, a snare is attached to the distal end of the metacarpal bone.
- With the help of two assistants, uniformly increasing force traction is applied on the snare (which is attached to the distal end of metacarpal bone).
- Due to this constantly increasing force traction, decorticated limb (skinless limb) is detached from the thorax and remove it.
- The digits or feet still attached to the skin, serve as a point of fixation for a traction cord in the final delivery of the foetus (see Fig. 26.2).

- In this way, the limb with the scapula is removed without crushing the maternal passage.
- **Generally the removal of one fore limb gives a sufficient reduction in the foetal diameter to allow delivery by force traction.**
- If delivery is not possible after this operation, the other fore leg must be removed in the same way.

CLINICAL POINTER

- Suppose, in anterior presentation, both forelimbs are equally accessible, it is no matter which is removed, but the right-handed operator will find it easier to perform foetotomy on the left fore leg of the calf and vice versa.
- This method can only be carried out successfully when the limb to be amputated projects from the vulva as far as the mid-metacarpal region. If other limb is also presented simultaneously, replace it in the uterus which provide more space for operation.

Hind limb :

- A skin incision is made on the medial aspect of the leg from fetlock joint to the under aspect of pelvis and the fingers are used for separation of skin (see Fig. 26.3).
- After disarticulating the fetlock joint, a wooden rod is inserted under the tendon Achilles and fixed by a 'finger of eight cord' (see Fig. 26.4).
- The hip joint is disarticulated by rotation and traction of wooden rod and the decorticated limb is withdrawn from the pelvis.

CLINICAL POINTER

In emergency where more sophisticated instruments are not available, removal of a hind limb or fore limb by the subcutaneous method can be performed with the simplest equipment, such as with any finger-knife. A skin incision is made on the medial aspect of the leg, from the fetlock joint to the under aspect of the pelvis (in case of hind limb) or to the scapula (in case of fore limb) and the fingers are used for separation of skin. The muscles connecting the femur to the trunk and pelvis (hind limb) or scapula to the thorax (fore limb) are divided, as far as possible, with finger's knife.

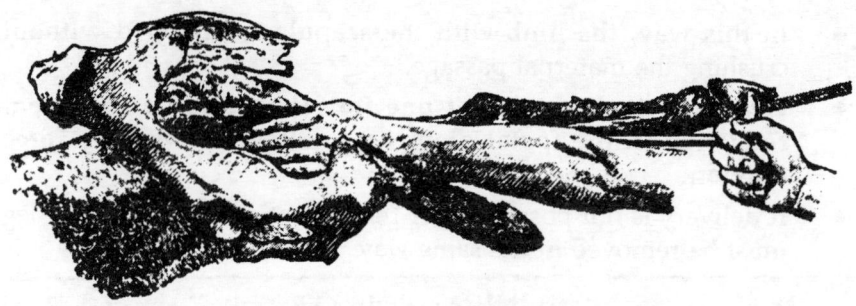

Fig. 26.3 : Subcutaneous amputation of the normally placed hind limb. Separation of the skin and muscles using Keller's spatula controlled by the hand. (Courtesy of Benesch, F. and Wright, J.G. 2001. Veterinary Obstetrics. Greenworld Publishers).

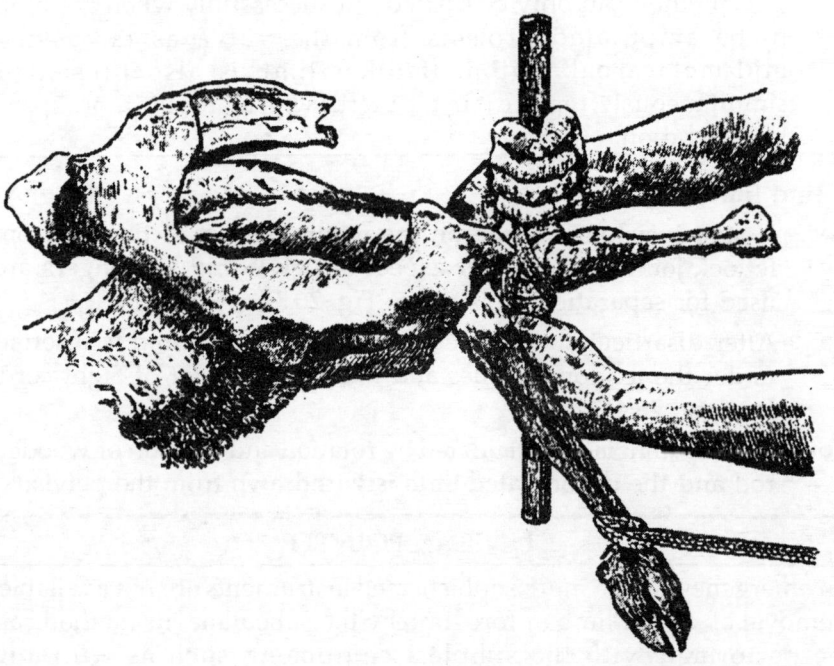

Fig. 26.4 : Subcutaneous amputation of the normally placed hind limb. The hip joint is disarticulated by torsion. The other limb is repelled as far as possible. The phalanges in the skin serve for the fixation of a foot-snare. (Courtesy of Benesch, F. and Wright, J.G. 2001. Veterinary Obstetrics. Greenworld Publishers).

Percutaneous foetotomy :

Removal or division of certain parts of the foetus along with skin to reduce the size of foetus is called percutaneous foetotomy.

Technique of percutaneous foetotomy :

- For percutaneous foetotomy, generally Thygesen's foetotome is used.
- Epidural anaesthesia should be given before starting the foetotomy because it reduces or stops the straining.
- If relaxation of uterine musculature is required, **Clenbuterol** should be used.
- At least one person is required to restrain the patient and ideally two person to assist the obstetrician.
- The metal saw wire must be threaded through one or both the tubes of Thygesen's foetotome before use according to conditions.
- If, the foetal part to be sectioned (cut) is directly accessible (eg. the head of a calf in normal anterior presentation) **both the tubes should be threaded**.
- If the foetal part to be sectioned is not directly accessible, then only one tube of the foetotome is threaded. The other end of wire is attached to the **introducer** which is passed around the part (to be cut) and pulled out from the birth canal and then passed through the other tube of foetotome.
- Placement of wire is always facilitated by generous use of obstetrical lubricant. About 2 litres or more of lubricant should be applied into the uterus.
- After fixing the loop around the foetus to be cut, tightly pull the wire.
- **A deep incision is made** at this position with knife to accommodate the wire.
- At this stage, the obstetrician should carefully check the position.
- Now, sawing is started by an assistant using **initially short strokes, then long strokes** and foetotome is held firmly in position by the obstetrician.
- Initially the wire takes a little more time to engage in the skin of the part so short sawing strokes should be used at this stage.
- Muscle is readily sawn but more effort is required for bone.

163

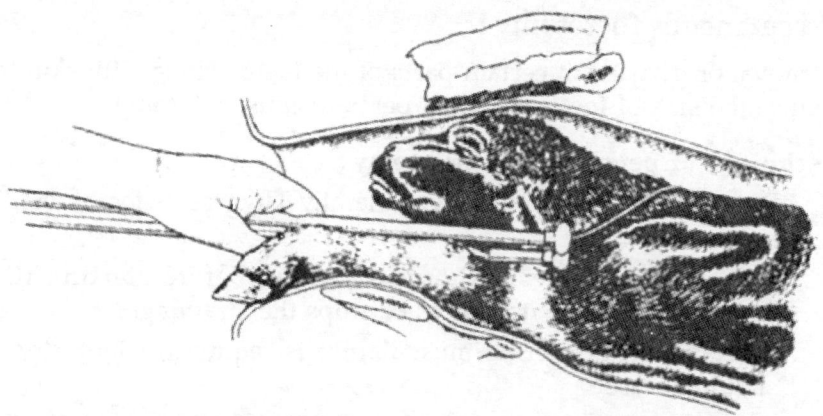

Fig. 26.5 : Foetotomy - Removal of head. Loop of foetotomy wire is over the head and neck along the base of the neck. (Courtesy of Jackson, P.G.G. 1995. Handbook of Veterinary Obstetrics. W.B. Saunders Company Limited).

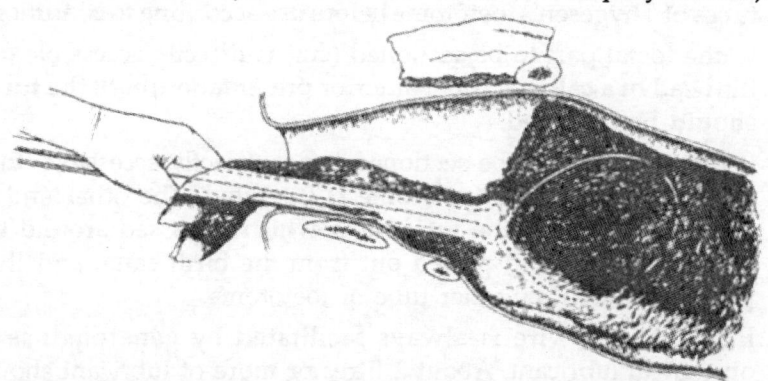

Fig. 26.6 : Foetotomy - Removal of a fore leg. A loop of foetotomy wire is passed along the leg to be removed. The foetotome is kept on the medial side of leg (dotted lines show medial side of leg). (Courtesy of Jackson, P.G.G. 1995. Handbook of Veterinary Obstetrics. W.B. Saunders Company Limited).

- The efficiency of sawing is increased, if the part is kept in tension by force traction.
- Once the foetal part has been cut, the wire will suddenly encounter much less resistance.
- The foetotome is then removed and the sectioned foetal part is retrieved and removed.
- **Great care must be taken during removal of part to ensure that birth canal is not damaged by sharp bony fragments.**
- An attempt is now made to deliver the calf by traction.

164

Complete foetotomy in anterior presentation :

(i) **Removal of the head :**

- **If head is protruding from the vulva** – attach rope to the head and simply cut the head with a knife or scalpel.

- **If head is within vagina :** Fix the loop of foetotomy wire over the base of the neck and then saw as close to the shoulder as possible (see Fig. 26.5).

(ii) **Removal of fore legs :** Fix the loop of foetotomy wire over the top of scapula of the leg to be removed and then saw the foreleg (see Fig. 26.6). After removing the head and one fore leg, an attempt should be made to deliver the calf by traction. If birth is not yet possible, remove the second leg also.

(iii) **Transverse division of thorax :** The thorax of the calf is removed by sawing the body across the **caudal to the ribs in the lumbar region (see Fig. 26.7).**

(iv) **Removal of abdominal viscera :** After removal of thorax, foetal abdominal viscera become exposed and is removed manually foetus.

(v) **Longitudinal division of pelvis :** Now the rear end of the foetus is inside the uterus after removal of the thorax. Divide the pelvic girdle longitudinally so that the caudal part of the foetus may be removed in two smaller parts **(see Fig. 26.8)**. Sectioning of pelvis is helped by holding it in position through self-tightening hooks **(Krey-Schottler's hook).**

Complete foetotomy in posterior presentation :

Removal of hind limbs :

- The foetotome instrument is threaded and the wire-loop is placed over one foot and passed over the limb so that the end of the loop lies anterior and medial to the wing of foetal ilium.

- Now, the head of instrument is placed lateral to the anus, and the tail of the calf must be included in the loop. This prevents the wire to slip down the leg (see Fig. 26.9).

- After fixing the loop, sawing is started and the severed limb is removed.

- If delivery is still impossible, the other hind limb must be removed and the fetus should be withdrawn as far as possible.

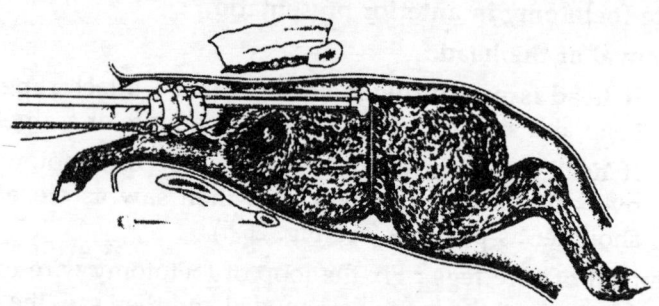

Fig. 26.7 : Foetotomy - Removal of thorax. The loop is placed just caudal to the last rib in the lumbar region. Transverse division through the trunk after removal of the head and fore limb. Note that sectioning of the thorax is helped by holding it in position by applying traction to it through a part of self-tightening hooks (Krey-Schottler's hooks). (Courtesy of Jackson, P.G.G. 1995. Handbook of Veterinary Obstetrics. W.B. Saunders Company Limited).

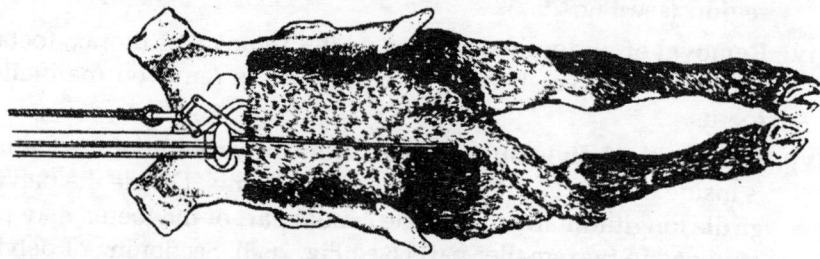

Fig. 26.8 : Longitudinal division of pelvis. Note that longitudinal division is helped by holding the hind parts in position by applying traction through self-tightening hooks (Krey-Schottler's hooks). (Courtesy of Jackson, P.G.G. 1995. Handbook of Veterinary Obstetrics. W.B. Saunders Company Limited).

Transverse division of trunk :

- If delivery is still impossible, then its trunk must be bisected by means of the wire loop.

Longitudinal division of anterior part of body :

- One or if necessary both forelimbs are amputed by passing the wire between neck and fore limb.

Advantages of foetotomy :

1. It reduces the size of the foetus.
2. It avoides caesarean operation.
3. It require little assistance.
4. It prevents possible trauma or injury to the dam during use of excessive force traction.

Disadvantages of foetotomy :

1. It may be dangerous, cause injuries or lacerations to the uterus or birth canal by instruments or sharp edges of bones.

2. The process may be time-taking and exhausting for both the dam and the operator.

3. It may be dangerous to the veterinarian by wound from instruments.

4. If the foetus is emphysematous, there is a possibility of infection to the operator's arm.

Note : *However, the advantages outweigh the disadvantages and foetotomy in large animals is a practical and successful way of relieving dystocia.*

To perform complete foetotomy in anterior and posterior presentation, following cuts are required :

Anterior Presentation :

No. of cuts	Parts to be amputated	Position of the wire saw	Position of the foetotome
1st cut	Head	Around the neck	Posterior part of the mandible
2nd cut	First fore limb	Between elbow joint & chest	Near scapula
3rd cut	Second forelimb	-do-	-do-
4th cut (Transverse division of thorax)	Posterier part of the chest	At right angle of foetotome head around foetus	Posterior of last foetal rib dorsally
5th cut (Longitudinal division of pelvis)	Pelvis bisection	In between tail & tuber ischii	Just cranial to the tuber coxae of the limb

Posterior presentation :

No. of cuts	Parts to be amputated	Position of saw wire	Position of the foetotome
1st cut	First hind limb	Between tuber ischium and tail head.	Near trochantor.
2nd cut	Second hind limb	-do-	-do-
3rd cut	Transverse division of foetal trunk (lumbar area)	At right angle to foetotome head around the foetus	Just caudal to foetal rib.
4th cut	Diagonal longitudinal division of fore-part.	Neck and fore limb on side and medial to opposite limb	Posterior to scapular attachment

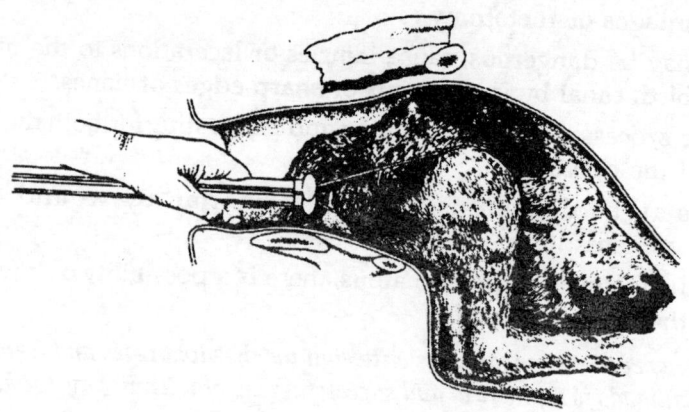

Fig. 26.9 : Removal of a hind limb with irreducible hip flexion (Breech presentation). (Courtesy of Jackson, P.G.G. 1995. Handbook of Veterinary Obstetrics. W.B. Saunders Company Limited).

Foetotomy versus Caesareaon operation:

- Foetotomy should be considered when the foetus is dead but caesarean section is considered when foetus is either dead or live.

- The obstetrician must decide which of these two techniques to use.

- For example, suppose, if a moderately sized foetus has a lateral deviation of the head, which cannot be manually corrected, and the birth canal is sufficiently dilated for the obstetrician to gain easy access to the base of the foetal neck, then foetotomy is indicated. In this condition, the foetal neck is sectioned (cut) and removed by force traction.

- If the foetus is in the same maldisposition as above but the cervix is only partially dilated making access to the foetus extremely difficult. In such circumstances, caesarean section is best option even though the foetus is dead.

- It has been suggested that foetotomy should ideally **not involve more than six cuts or take more than an hour to complete**. If it ˙ is thought that these limits cannot be **fullfilled** then caesarean section provides an alternative option.

- The inexperienced obstetrician may suggests the more familiar technique of caesarean section, although **the prognosis of this technique is poorer when the foetus is dead.**

- **In some circumstances, there may be no alternative to foetotomy.**

For example, in some cases, the calving has been unattended and the dead foetus is found with its head and part of the thorax protruding from the vagina. It cannot be delivered by traction because of **stifle lock** and it can not be repelled into the uterus so that caesarean section can be performed. Foetotomy provides the only solutions in this condition.

- **Caesarean section is indicated over foetotomy if the foetus is alive and the owner wants to save the foetus.**
- **Caesarean section is more difficult to perform successfully in the mare** than the other domestic animals. Therefore, foetotomy or force traction is method of choice in this species.
- The genital tract of the mare is more easily traumatized than that of the cow. Therefore foetotomy should be performed carefully and gently.
- If after 10 minutes of judicious traction no progress is made, the obstetrician must decide to a caesarean operation if the calf is alive or dead, or foetotomy if the calf is dead. **There are many cases where it is difficult to assess whether a calf is live or dead, in that condition, the calf should be given the benefit of doubt.**

Some terminology used in foetotomy operation :
- **Decapitation :** It is the separation of head at the atlantlo-occipital joint.
- **Decollation :** It is the separation of neck at the greatest curvature (i.e. the base of neck).
- **Cephalotomy :** Reducing the size of cranium by simple puncture, incision or crushing of the cranial envelope.
- **Detruncation :** Division of body.
- **Evisceration (eventration) :** The process by which the volume of thoracic and abdominal cavity is reduced by removing their organs.

OBSERVATIONS :

Date ....

- Case No. ....
- Species ....
- Breed ....

169

- Age ....
- Parity ....
- History ...:..........................
- Presentation ....
- Position ....
- Posture ....
- Foetus   *live/dead*
- Any abnormality in foetus ....
- Condition of dam ....
- Type of foetotomy used ....
- Instruments used ....
- Time taken ....
- Pre-operative and post-operative treatment given.

Rx.

1.

2.

3.

4.

EXERCISE :

1.   Practice foetotomy operation in dummy calf in phantom box.

2.   In which species, foetotomy is most commonly used ?

Ans.

3.   In which species, foetotomy is almost never used ?

Ans.

4.   During subcutaneous foetotomy, rope is fixed around the pastern joint instead of fetlock joint. Why ?

Ans.

5.   Suppose, during subcutaneous foetotomy, both fore legs are equally accessible, which leg will you prefer to perform foetotomy and why?

Ans.

6.   Can subcutaneous foetotomy be performed, if legs are inside the vagina. Give reason.

Ans.

7. How can epidural anaesthesia help in foetotomy ?

Ans.

8. What is the use of clenbuterol in foetotomy ?

Ans.

9. Write the dose of clenbuterol in cattle.

Ans.

10. If the foetal part to be sectioned is not directly accessible,then initially only one tube of the foetotome is threaded.Why ?

Ans.

11. Why a deep incision is made at the point of position of saw-wire ?

Ans.

12. Why great care must be taken during removal of sectioned foetal part ?

Ans.

13. What is the site of transverse division of thorax ?

Ans.

14. What is the site of longitudinal division of pelvis ?

Ans.

15. What is the use of Krey Schottler's hook during foetotomy ?

Ans.

16. Why tail of calf is included during the amputation of hind limb in posterior presentation?

Ans.

17. How many maximum cuts can be given during foetotomy ?

Ans.

❈ ❈ ❈ ❈ ❈

If all the flowers which blossom should become fruit, there would be no room on the Earth for them.

Chapter 27

Techniques of Caesarean Section in Farm Animals

MATERIALS REQUIRED :

- Appropriate drugs for sedation and local anaesthesia
- Resuscitation facilities including arrangements to dry and warm the calf. **Doxapram hydrochloride (50 mg) may be kept ready in a syringe with a suitable needle prior to surgery because sometimes, it is needed urgently when calf is delivered.**
- Sterilized calving ropes or chains which may be needed during removal of the foetus from the uterus.
- Antiseptic solution for skin preparation – 7.5% Povidone-iodine or 4% Chlorhexidin gluconate and surgical spirit.
- Sterilized drape.
- Surgical kit : Scalpel, rat-toothed forceps, scissors, six haemostats, needle-holders, round-body and cutting suture needles.
- Suture material.
- Antibiotics : Strepto-penicillin or ampicillin is useful.

Caesarean section : *The delivery of the foetus usually at parturition by laparohysterotomy is called caesarean section.* The word caesarean is said to derive either from an edict by Julius Caesar that woman was about to die in advanced child birth and this operation was performed to save the child or from the Latin word *caeso matris utera* means cutting of mother's uterus.

Indications :

- **Foetopelvic disproportion,** including cases of **misalliance** and post maturity.
- **Foetal maldisposition,** which cannot be corrected by manipulation.

- **Irreducible uterine torsion.**
- **Incomplete dialatation of cervix** or other parts of birth canal.
- **Foetal monsters,** which cannot be delivered by other means.
- **Uterine rupture** or severe uterine haemorrhage.
- **Foetal emphysema.**
- **Mummification and hydroallantois** after failure of induction of parturition by drugs.
- **Bicornual pregnancy** in mares.
- Pregnancy toxaemia in ewes and does.
- Rupture of prepubic tendon.

Selection of operative site :

Large animals :

The sites are
      (i) Left flank.
      (ii) Right flank.
      (iii) Ventro-lateral.
      (iv) Ventral or mid line.

Small animals :

The sites are
      (i) Flank region with an oblique angle parallel to the last rib.
      (ii) Midline or linea alba.

The advantages and disadvantages of the various sites may be summarized as :

Advantages of flank laparotomy
• Only local anaesthesia is required.
• The incision may be easily extended if necessary.
• Risk of postoperative soiling of wound or herniation is less.
• It may be performed on the standing or laterally recumbent cow.
• Easier correction of uterine torsion.
• Finally, wound dehiscence is more **manageable** as compared with lower abdominal incisions.

Disadvantages of flank laparotomy
• The uterus is often difficult to exteriorize prior to opening.
• The peritoneum is readily contaminated with uterine contents especially if the calf is dead and/or emphysematous.

Left flank laparotomy :
- The risk of small intestine coming out from the site of wound is negligible (**merit**).
- The rumen may cause **hindrance** to access of the uterus (**demerit**).

Right flank laparotomy :
- Allow good access to a calf in the right uterine horn (**merit**).
- The risk of the small intestine to come out from the laparotomy wound is higher (**demerit**).

Ventro-lateral laparotomy :
- A ventro lateral incision is particularly indicated **for the removal of an emphysematous foetus.**
- · The cow should be in right lateral recumbency for ventro-lateral laparotomy.
- The advantage of this approach is that it gives good exposure of the uterus.
- Another advantage is, it **minimizes the risk of contamination from uterine contents** to the abdominal cavity or peritoneum.

Disadvantages :
- **Repair of the abdominal muscle layers are more difficult** because the muscles remain under tension and sutures may tear the muscles.
- **Risk of post-operative soiling of wound is more.**

Midline or paramedian incision :
- It is not commonly used in the field condition because general anaesthesia or heavy sedation is required and respiratory function of the dam is compromised in this condition.
- **Risk of post operative soiling of wound or herniation is higher.**
- However this technique gives excellent access to the uterus.

• **Left flank incision is the most common technique and is most appropriate for the standing animal.**
• A right flank incision is uncommon; however, it is indicated if the left flank approach is obstructed by adhesion as a result of previous surgery.

Anaesthesia :

- Sedation should be avoided (if possible) because it can cause recumbency during surgery and may be detrimental to foetal survival.

- If sedation is necessary, xylazine is commonly used (0.05-0.1 mg/kg b.w. I/M).

Unfortunately, xylazine is an ecbolic (increase contraction of uterus), making surgery more difficult and cause ruminal bloat which can obstruct the access to the uterus.

- For flank incision, **paravertebral anaesthesia should be given.**

Paravertebral anaesthesia :

- Signs of successful densensitization are warm, hyperaemic and flaccid flank with no response to pain when tested with an 18 gauze needle.

- **Advantage of paravertebral anaesthesia** is that the whole flank musculature is desensitized and flaccid which facilitates exploration of the abdomen during surgery and closure of wound.

- **Disadvantage of paravertebral nerve block** is that vasodilatation occurs in muscle layers which causes a greater degree of haemorrhage during surgery.

- **Inverted - L block :**

An inverted - L block of the flank is an alternative to paravertebral anaesthesia.

- An 18-gauge needle is used to administer 2% lignocaine with adrenaline at several sites. The number of sites is dependent on the length of the proposed incision.

- At each point, 5 ml. of local anaesthetic is injected subcutaneously in each direction of the incision line and 10 ml. into musculature.

- **Peritoneum may not be effectively anaesthetized, causing reaction by the patient when it is incised (disadvantage).**

- However, this technique is quick and reliable and requires minimal training.

- **Epidural anaesthesia :**

Epidural anaesthesia is not essential but is useful to prevent straining and tail movement during surgery. Sometime it causes recumbency during surgery (demerit).

Pre-operative medication :
- Pre-operative antibiotic is strongly recommended.
- Tocolytic agents such as clenbuterol hydrochloride (10 ml) should be administered by intramuscular or intravenous route.

Surgical technique :

The surgical technique is performed in following steps:
1. Opening of the flank
2. Locating the uterus
3. Opening of the uterus
4. Removal of the foetus
5. Management of the placenta
6. Closing of the uterine incision
7. Closing of the laparotomy incision

Opening of the flank :
- An incision is made through the skin 25-30 cm. in length approximately 10 cm. below the transverse process of the lumbar vertebrae and half-way between the last rib and the tuber coxae.
- Check bleeding at every step.
- Before opening the peritoneum, the haemostats are used to control bleeding points in the muscle layers which should be removed after ligating the vessels.
- Incise the peritoneum.

Locating the uterus :
- The uterus lies caudal to and below the rumen.
- If uterus is not visible, then it is searched by pushing the rumen forward.

Opening of the uterus :
- The opening should be made over the foetal extremity in the greater curvature of the pregnant uterine horn.
- The incision should be approximately 20 cm. long in the direction of the longitudinal muscles and in between the cotyledons, otherwise profuse haemorrhage may occur.

Removal of the foetus :

- If the foetus in anterior presentation, **then removed rear end of foetus first at caesarean** section and if the foetus is in posterior presentation, **then remove front end.**

Management of placenta :

- If the placenta is easily and quickly detachable, it should be carefully removed from the uterus.
- If not, it should be left in the site **even when the cervix is closed.**
- Furea bolus is kept in the uterus.

Closing of the uterine incision :

- Uterine incision is cleaned with saline and closed with Cushing and Lambert sutures by using chromic catgut No.1 or 0.

Closing of the laparotomy incision :

- Before the closure of the incision, a quantity of crystalline penicillin or ampicillin (1-2 gm) may be instilled into the abdomen as a soluble solution to minimize the risk of peritoneal infection.
- Abdominal incision is closed in routine manner.

Post operative care :

1. Routine antibiotic cover (with strepto-penicillin for 5-7 days).
2. Fluid therapy.
3. Regular dressing of wound.

Complications of caesarean section
• Peritonitis
• Wound breakdown
• Seroma formation – A pocket of sterile serous fluid accumulates between muscle layers or under the skin. This can be confirmed when a sterile needle is inserted — serum flow-out.
• Retention of the foetal membranes
• Metritis
• Infertility
• Mastitis (*E. coli* infection)
• Sudden death.

OBSERVATIONS :

Date : ....

- Case No. ....
- Species ....
- Breed ....
- History
  (a) Age of dam ....
  (b) Gestation period   *short/prolonged*
  (c) Breed of sire ....
  (d) Others ....
- Duration of dystocia ....
- Nature of dystocia ....
- Physical condition of dam ....
- Mucus membrane ....
- Genital discharge ....
- Condition of cervix ....
- Size of foetus ....
- Any abnormality of the foetus ....
- Whether handled by other ....
- **Clinical parameters :**
  Temperature ....
  Respiration rate ....
  Pulse rate ....
  Rumen motility ....
  Degree of dehydration ....
- Restraining method ....
- Systemic anaesthesia (if any) ....
- Local anaesthetics ....
- Type of nerve block ....
- Pre-operative treatment ....
- Treatment during operation ....
- Foetus .... live/dead
- Condition of foetus ....
- Post operative complication (if any) ....
- Post operative condition of dam ....

- **Post operative treatment.**

Rx.

    1.

    2.

    3.

    4.

EXERCISE :

1. Which site should be selected for delivery of dead emphysematous calf ?

Ans.

2. In which condition right flank caesarean section is recommended for delivery of foetus ?

Ans.

3. In which approach, abdominal wound is closed with interrupted non-absorbable suture and why ?

Ans.

4. What is the site of skin incision in ventro-lateral approach ?

Ans.

5. What is the site of skin incision in midline approach ?

Ans.

6. What is the site of incision on the uterus ?

Ans.

7. Why incision on the uterus is given in between the row of cotyledons?

Ans.

8. When incision on the uterus is required to extend then in which direction incision should be extended and why ?

Ans.

9. What is the limitation of inverted L-block ?

Ans.

10. Which drug is given after caesarean section to neutralize the effect of clenbuterol ?

Ans.

� � � � �

> *Success is the child of two very plain parents – punctuality and accuracy.*
> *– O.S. Marden*

Chapter **28**

Diagnosis and Management of Uterine Torsion in Farm Animals

Uterine torsion : *Rotation of uterus on its long axis is called uterine torsion.*

Incidence :
- Most common in cattle and buffalo
- Occasionally in mare, ewe, doe and bitch.
- Rare in sow
- Breed - more in **surti** than other buffalo breeds due to wallowing habit.
- More common in pluriparous animals.

Etiology :
1. The bovine pregnant uterus has been said to be basically unstable for a number of reasons.
   - The lesser curvature of the uterus in advanced pregnancy is supported dorso laterally by the broad ligament whereas the greater curvature lies free in the abdominal cavity.
   - The cranial parts of the uterine horns lie on the abdominal floor with no stabilizing ligament attachment.
   - A calf occupies only one horn of the uterus, making the uterine horn heavier and more bulky on one side than other that increase instability of uterus.
   - These anatomical arrangements described above together with the manner in which a cow lies down and gets up predispose torsion. She goes down on knee first while sitting and elevates her hind quarter first before getting up. A slight fall or slip during this time or even a butt by a neighbouring cow may predispose to torsion in bovine.

- Attachment of amnion : Partial attachment of amniotic sac to the chorioallantois in bovine predisposes torsion of uterus as a result of violent foetal movement.
2. Confinement in stables for longer period.
3. Hilly region.
4. Malnutrition – causes weakness of ligaments and lack of uterine tone.

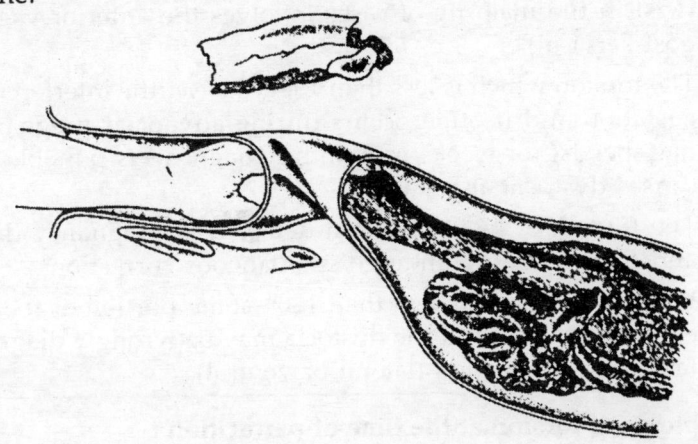

Fig. 28.1 : Torsion of the uterus - Vaginal examination. Note that vaginal examination reveals an abnormal disposition of the birth canal. The hand cannot be immediately passed anteriorly towards the cervix. The vagina narrows conically and folds indicate the direction of trosion. If the torsion is less than 180 degree, the obstetrician's hand may be passed through the constriction to palpate the foetus. If torsion is greater than 180 degree, the birth canal may be totally occluded with the vagina coming to a conical end with no recognizable cervix being palpable. (Courtesy of Jackson, P.G.G. 1995. Handbook of Veterinary Obstetrics. W.B. Saunders Company Limited).

Degree of torsion :

Degrees	Rotation of uterus
1st degree –	90^0
2nd degree –	180^0 – ½
3rd degree –	270^0 – ¾
4th degree	360^0 – complete.

Direction of torsion :

- Clockwise or right torsion.
- Anti-clockwise or left torsion.

Right torsion is more common.

Site of torsion :

- Pre-cervical (posterior part of uterine body).
- Post-cervical (anterior vagina).

INTERESTING FACTS
<ul><li>Although the uterus rotates aboutits longitudinal axis, the actual twist in the majority of cases involves the anterior vagina (i.e. post cervical).</li><li>The torsion which is less than 180^0 causes little interference with gestation and it often occurs during advanced pregnancy and may persist for weeks or months. Diagnosis is possible when it causes dystocia at term.</li><li>The torsion of $45\text{-}90^0$ is often detected at pregnancy diagnosis and they probably undergo spontaneous correction.</li><li>When the torsion is less than 180^0 some portion of foetus may enter the vagina and the dystocia may be wrongly diagnosed as faulty foetal position (lateral or ventral).</li></ul>

Symptoms of torsion at the time of parturition :

Uterine torsion is a complication of **late first stage or early second stage labour.**

- The first sign may be noted towards the end of the first stage of labour, which is prolonged and the cow shows signs of mild discomfort (uneasy, restless, colic, kicking and switching its tail).
- Tenesmus or abdominal straining characteristic of the second stage of labour but it is either absent or mild in uterine torsion.

CLINICAL POINTER
An owner complains that his/her cow was showing the symptoms of parturition from the last 8 to 18 hours or more but true labour or straining has not occurred. Such a history of a prolonged first stage of parturition is usually observed in uterine torsion.

- Tachycardia
- Anorexia
- The patient may adopt a **"rocking horse" stance** so that dorsal surface of her spine is concave and the fore limbs and hind limb are held respectively forward and backward than normal.

- If the twist is of 90-180°,
    - Discharge comes from vagina
    - Water bag may come out and limbs of the foetus may be in the pelvic cavity.
- If the twist is of 360°, the vaginal passage becomes narrower and the cervix cannot be palpated through vagina.

Symptoms of torsion during gestation period :

- If mild (45-90°) – No symptoms.
- If 180° or more :
    - Abdominal pain
    - Anorexia
    - Constipation
    - Lack of rumination
    - Rapid pulse rate.
- Late pregnancy and severe case :
    - Complete anorexia
    - Foetid diarrhoea
    - Suspended rumination
    - Rapid pulse rate
    - Normal to sub-normal temperature
    - Difficulty in micturition due to involvement of urinary bladder
    - Foetus dies and becomes emphysematous
    - Shock, collapse and death may occur within 24-72 hours.

CLINICAL POINTER
The symptoms of torsion during gestation period may be confused with traumatic gastritis, indigestion, pyelonephritis or intestinal intussusception. A cow over 6 months pregnancy if showing above symptoms, should be subjected to rectal examination.

Diagnosis :

1) By history
2) By symptoms
3) Vaginal examination (see Fig. 28.1) :
- If the hand is inserted into vagina, it cannot be passed easily towards cervix.

- Twisting of hand indicates whether torsion is clockwise or anti-clockwise.
- Intensity of twisting or stenosis of birth canal indicates severity of torsion.
- Birth-canal is narrow and stenosed in the region of anterior vagina.
- **If the torsion is greater than 180^0, it is usually impossible to pass the hand through the twisted portion of the birth canal.**
- **If the torsion is less than 180^0, the obstetrician's hand may be passed through the birth canal to palpate the foetus.**
- **Dorsal commissure of the vulva is pulled forward and left in** case of **left torsion** and **forward and right** in case of **right torsion** (270^0 to 360^0).

Treatment :
(1) Rolling of dam
(2) Schaffer's method
(3) Rotation of foetus and uterus through the birth canal
(4) Abdominal ballotment
(5) Stimulation of vigorous foetal movement
(6) Suspending the cow's body by her hocks
(7) Laparotomy
(8) Caesarean section

1) Rolling of dam (see Fig. 28.2) :
- Sedative (Siquil 5 ml IM) should be administered.
- The udder should be emptied.`
- Ascertain the side of torsion.
- **Cast the animal in lateral recumbency on the same side as the direction of the torsion.**
- The front and the hind limbs are secured **separately.**
- Keep hand in birth canal and grasp the foetal part (if cervix is dilated).
- Roll the cow in the same direction of torsion.
- After the cow has been rolled through 180^0, her body must be pushed slowly over the legs and sternum to bring back the same position to continue the rolling in the same direction.

- Examine the vaginal passage to find out whether rolling is effective or not. If the rolling is effective, the spiral folds and stenosis of birth canal starts to disappear. If the rolling is in wrong direction, vaginal folds become more tight.

- After each two or three rapid rotations of the cow's body, the birth-canal should be examined.

- **Occasionally, there may be a rush of foetal fluids from the uterus as the torsion is relieved.**

- **After correction of uterus, the foetus should be pulled out by applying forced traction as soon as possible because the cervix**

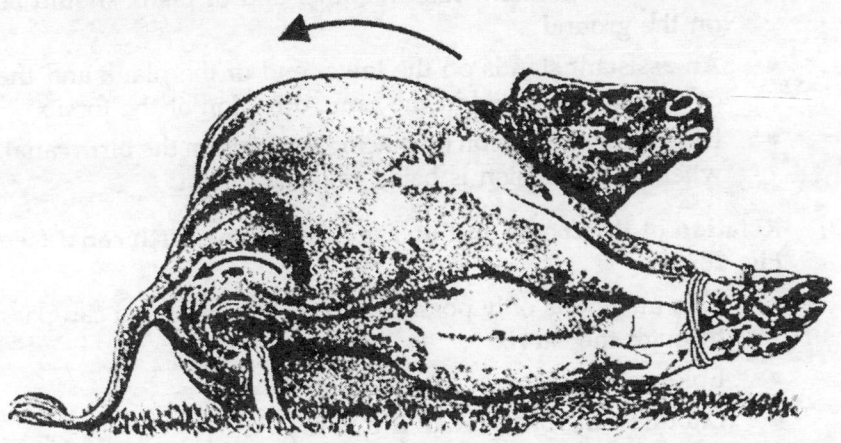

Fig. 28.2 : Torsion of the uterus-rolling the cow (Courtesy of Jackson, P.G.G. 1995. Handbook of Veterinary Obstetrics. W.B. Saunders Company Limited).

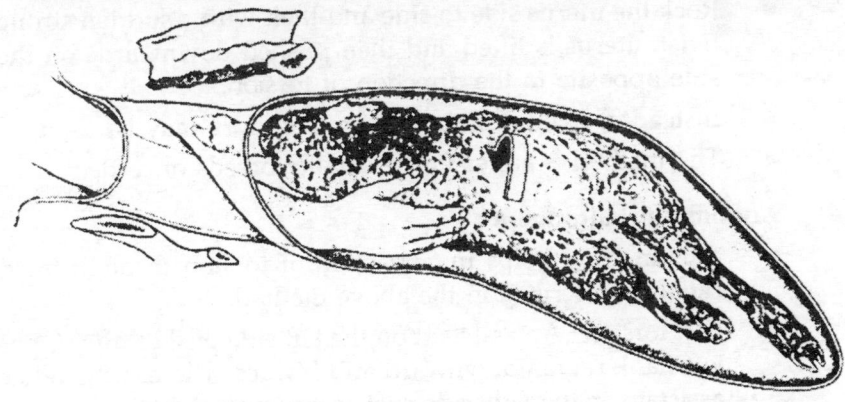

Fig. 28.3 : Torsion of the uterus-rolling of the foetus and uterus *per vaginum* (Courtesy of Jackson, P.G.G. 1995. Handbook of Veterinary Obstetrics. W.B. Saunders Company Limited).

may close within 30 minutes of correction of torsion which prevents foetal delivery by the vaginal route.

2) **Schaffer's method :**

It is a modification of rolling method.

- The cow is casted on the same side as the direction of torsion.
- The legs are tied in the same manner as in the above method.
- A plank 9 to 12 feet long and 8 to 12 inches wide is placed over the abdomen while the other end of plank should be on the ground.
- An assistant stands on the lower end of the plank and the cow is slowly rolled in the same direction of the torsion.
- Determine the torsion by placing the hand in the birth canal, whether the torsion is being relieved or not.

3) **Rotation of the foetus and uterus through the birth canal (see Fig. 28.3) :**

- This method is only possible if obstetrician's hand can pass through the cervix.
- Epidural anaesthesia should be given.
- Lubricate the birth canal, if it is dry.
- The foetus is grasped by a convenient prominence such as elbow, sternum or thigh.
- Rock the uterus side to side and then with a sudden strong twist, uterus is lifted and then pushed downwards on the side opposite to the direction of torsion.
- Instead of hand, Cammerer's torsion fork may be used.
- The method is easier in the smaller breeds of cattle.

4) **Abdominal ballotment :**

- This method helps in correction of torsion through birth canal as described in the above method.
- Left torsion : An assistant on the left side pushes the upper left flank region downward and inward whereas the other assistant on the right side pushes the lower right flank region upward and inward.
- Right torsion : Upper right flank – Push downward and inward.

Lower left flank – push upward and inward.

- Both the assistants should push alternatively at regular intervals in quick succession which causes the uterus to roll from side to side and this helps the operator working via birth-canal.

5) **Stimulation of vigorous foetal movement :**
   - This method helps other manual methods of correction of torsion.
   - The hand is passed in the uterus, and eye ball of the foetus is pressed firmly. This results in strong reflex movement of the foetus that may aid in manual correction of the torsion.

6) **Suspending the cow's body by her hock :**
   - It is an old and crude technique. Therefore, it is not recommended.
   - The gravid uterus rotates more easily into its normal position, when a cow is hanged.

7) **Laparotomy :**
   - If the case cannot be corrected by either of the above methods, a laparotomy should be performed on the standing cow through the left or right sublumbar fossa.
   - Caesarean section may be required if after correction of torsion, the cervix remain closed. **Therefore, left flank approach is preferable.**

Left torsion :
- After performing laparotomy, the hand is passed between the uterus and the left flank until it touches the abdominal floor and the foetal part is held through the uterine wall.
- Rock the uterus by lifting and lowering and finally lifting the uterus in rotating manner upward and push it to the right side.

Right torsion :
- The hand is passed over and down between the uterus and right flank, and the foetal part is held through the uterine wall.
- Rock the uterus in the same manner as above.
- Finally lift the uterus upward strongly in rotating manner and push it to left side.

8) Caesarean section :

It is indicated when correction by laparotomy or other means fails or cervix is insufficiently dilated.

Sheep and goat :

Uterine torsion is corrected by hanging the body.

OBSERVATIONS :

Date ....

- Case No. ....
- Species ....
- Breed ....
- Age ....
- History ....
- Degree of torsion ....
- Direction of torsion ....
- Site of torsion ....
- Symptoms` ...., ..., ...,
................., ..., ..., ...,
...................,
- Method of correction of torsion applied ....
- Condition of foetus ....
- Condition of dam ....
- Post – operative treatment (if given any)

Rx.

1.

2.

3.

4.

EXERCISE :

1. Why uterine torsion is uncommon in mare?

Ans.

2. Tenesmus or abdominal straining is characteristics of the second stage of labour but it is absent or mild in case of uterine torsion. Why ?

Ans.

3.   Why forelegs and hindlegs should not be tied together during the rolling of dam for correction of uterine torsion?

Ans.

4.   Rolling of dam should be in the same direction and rapidly for the correction of uterine torsion. Give reason.

Ans.

5.   How many assistants are required for rolling of dam ?

Ans.

6.   In Schaffer's method, less assistance is required in comparison to typical rolling method. Give reason.

Ans.

7.   What is the principle of Schaffer's method for the correction of uterine torsion ?

Ans.

8.   In which condition laparotomy is indicated for the correction of uterine torsion ?

Ans.

9.   What is the logic behind the rolling of dam to correct the uterine torsion ?

Ans.

10.   What is the peculiar style of cow to lies down and get up ?

Ans.

11.   Which torsion is common, pre-cervical or post-cervical ?

Ans.

12.   Why foetid dirrhoea is found in severe case of uterine torsion in late pregnancy ?

Ans.

❊   ❊   ❊   ❊   ❊

You are more successful than you realize.

PART – III

CURRENT DRUG THERAPY

Special features :

- 'New Zealand Method' for replacement of prolapsed mass.
- Discussions on efficacy of different antimicrobial agents on female genital tract.
- Selection of most appropriate drugs for therapy.
- 'Artificial Induction of Lactation' in cattle.
- Effects of **homoeopathic drugs** on female genital tracts.
- **Collagenase therapy** – A new approach for the treatment of RFM.
- Arguments against and in favour of manual removal of RFM.
- Synergistic activities of *A. pyogenes*, *Fusobacterium* and *Bacteroid* spp.
- NEFA
- **Night and Clenbuterol.**

Chapter 29

Diagnosis and Therapeutic Management of Anoestrus Cow

Definition :

"Anoestrus is a broad term that indicates the lack of oestrus expression at an expected time".

Classification :

(A) On the basis of corpus luteum (CL)

(i) **Presence of functional corpus luteum (functional anoestrus or apparent anoestrus).**
- Anoestrus due to pregnancy.
- Anoestrus due to pyometra.
- Anoestrus due to mummified foetus.
- Anoestrus due to macerated foetus.
- Silent heat or weak heat.

(ii) **Absence of functional corpus luteum (true anoestrus)**

The ovaries are quiescent, inactive and do not have any functional CL, This condition is referred to as true anoestrus. This may be due to :
- Malnutrition.
- Lactational stress.
- Seasonal stress.
- Chronic wasting disease.
- Senility.

(B) **On the basis of stage of the animal :**

1. **Prepubertal anoestrus**
- Delayed puberty – due to undernutrition.

193

- Abnormal reproductive tract – Freemartins, hermaphrodites, segmental aplasia of paramesonephric duct and ovarian hypoplasia.
- Debilitating disease such as chronic pneumonia etc.

Note : *A heifer must attain approximately two-third of its adult size before the attainment of puberty.*

2. **Postpartum anoestrus :**
- **Physiological anoestrus** for 2-3 weeks after parturition.
- **Lactational stress.**
- **Nutritional effects** such as negative energy balance and deficiency of micro nutrients.
- **Uterine diseases** such as RFM, metritis, pyometra etc.
- **Chronic debilitating diseases** such as leg injuries, displaced abomasum or hardware disease.

3. **Post service anoestrus :**
- Pregnancy.
- Pyometra.
- Luteal cyst.
- Silent oestrus.

Lactation and Anoestrus
The act of suckling stimulates the prolactin secretion which increase the period of anoestrus. It has been shown that suckling decreases LH secretion. This prevents the first postpartum ovulation and return of cyclicity. Plasma cortisol level increases in suckled cow which depresses LH secretion and sensitivity of pituitary gland to GnRH.

Treatment of true anoestrus :

1. Deworming with appropriate drug e.g. Albendazole, Fenbendazole etc.
2. Mineral mixture supplement action for one month.
3. Phosphorus injection (Tonophosphan) 10 ml. intramuscularly for three days.
4. Gentle ovarian massage and **painting of external os with Lugol's iodine** on alternate day three times.

DO YOU KNOW ?

Application of Lugol's iodine on the cervix causes local irritation and results in reflex stimulation of anterior pituitary for secretion of gonadotrophins and thus, cyclicity starts.

5.   If the above conventional treatments fail, then **herbal heat inducer drug** can be used for example Prajana, Sajani, Janova, Fertikit etc. Prajana Forte 2 capsule daily for three days orally. If she does not come in heat then repeat on 10th, 11th and 12th days.

6.   **CLOMIPHENE CITRATE** : (Fertivet, Clofert etc.) One tablet for five days orally. One tablet should be dissolved in 500 ml of water. Just before drenching the medicine, 125 ml 10% **Sodium bicarbonate** or 1% **Copper sulphate** should be drenched which **closes rumeno-reticular groove** so that the medicine directly goes to abomasum.

Depth of Anoestrus

Depth of anoestrus can be measured by per-rectal examination. The cow with very small, inactive ovaries, which are devoid of any significant structures (i.e. no palpable follicles or luteal tissue) are considered to be in greater depth of anoestrus than those large ovaries containing palpable follicles.

---

7.   **Hormonal therapy :**

(a) Administration of GnRH analogues :

Receptal (Buserelin 20 mg) 5 ml – I/M

CLINICAL POINTERS

●   The cows and heifers with completely smooth and non functional ovaries i.e. in deep anoestrus respond very poor. Therapy for these cows must be started after correcting the nutritional deficiency or systemic disease.

●   The cows and heifers which are in deep anoestrus, the administration of a single injection of GnRH may be ineffective in stimulation of ovulation. Therefore, second injection of GnRH 10 days later is necessary.

●   The calf removal for 48 hrs improve the ovulatory response by GnRH.

●   The GnRH analogues stimulate the oestrus within 1-3 weeks after treatment. This effect is probably not mediated through LH, but may involve a long-term stimulation of FSH secretion, which initiates follicular growth or development.

(b) Administration of eCG or PMSG :

- The most potent gonadotrophic drug that is available for use in cattle is equine chorionic gonadotropin (eCG).
- It can be used to stimulate ovarian activity and can induce follicular growth and oestrus within 2-5 days.
- Dose 1500 – 3000 IU I/M or I/V

Drawback of eCG
When eCG is administered at a dose rate of 3000 – 4500 IU, it causes superovulation rather than initiating normal ovarian activity. Therefore, it is not advised to inseminate in the induced oestrus but inseminate in next normal oestrus. But if the cow is not inseminated, there is possibility that she will relapse into anoestrus.

(c) Administration of progesterone :

Principle of progesterone administration
The mechanism behind this therapy is to mimic the luteal phase and sudden withdrawal of the progesterone to induce heat.

- Intramuscular oily preparation of progesterone injection (Duraprogen) does not give good result because it should be given daily for several days and also concentration does not decline suddenly at the end of treatment.
- Intravaginal route of administration of progesterone gives the most favourable result. **PRID or CIDR** device is placed in anoestrous cows for 7-14 days. Most cows show oestrus within few days of their removal. After removal of the device, sudden decline of progesterone occurs unlike duraprogen.
- Subcutaneous ear implant of **norgestomet** also gives good result.

(d) Oestrogens administration :

Oestrogens easily induce behavioural oestrus but no follicular growth or ovulation occurs.

Treatment of silent heat :

- Inject any one $PGF_2\alpha$ analogue when active CL remain present and do double AI after 48-72 hrs.

OBSERVATIONS :

Date ....

- Case No. ....

- Species ....
- Breed ....
- Age ....
- Number of calving.................................
- Date of last calving ....
- Any other history ....
- Per-rectal examination finding
  Ovary ....
  Uterus...

Treatment

    Rx

        1. ....
        2. ....
        3. ....
        4. ....

EXERCISE :

1. Define true anoestrus.

Ans.

2. Define apparent anoestrus.

Ans.

3. Define silent heat.

Ans.

4. Why dewormer should be given before starting the treatment of anoestrus ?

Ans.

5. What is the effect of ovarian massage in case of anoestrus ?

Ans.

6. What is the drawback of eCG treatment in case of anoestrus ?

Ans.

7. What is the drawback of intramuscular injection of oily preparation of progesterone in the treatment of anoestrus ?

Ans.

8.   What is the drawback of oestrogen treatment in inducing heat ?

Ans.

❋ ❋ ❋ ❋ ❋

> *Many of life's failures are people who did not realize how close they were to sucess when they gave up.*

Chapter **30**

Diagnosis and Therapeutic Management of Cystic Ovarian Degeneration

Definition : *"Ovarian cysts are defined as follicle like ovarian structures that are 2.5 cm. in diameter or larger and persist for 10 days or more generally in the absence of corpus luteum."*

OR

"Ovaries are said to be cystic when they contain one or more fluid-filled structures larger than a mature follicle (>2.5 cm. in diameter), which persist for more than 10 days and result in aberrant reproductive function."

Synonyms

Various synonyms are used for this disease which include 'cystic ovarian disease', 'cystic ovarian degeneration', 'cystic Graafian follicles', 'Ovarian cysts', 'luteal ovarian cysts' and 'cystic cows.'

Etiology :
- Deficiency of LH secretion during the pre-ovulatory stage.

INTERESTING FACT
This deficiency or failure of LH-release mechanism is not due to deficiency of GnRH but due to insensitivity of the hypothalamic-pituitary axis to elevated levels of oestradiol.

- There is also some evidence that ovarian cysts may be due to defect within the ovary. The ability of follicles to respond to the preovulatory LH surge is dependent upon the timely formation of LH receptors on its surface during follicular maturation. If less number of receptors are present on the follicle, it will result in ovulatory failure as well as cystic ovary.

199

Predisposing factors :

- **Hereditary predisposition :** Higher incidence in dairy breeds as compared to beef breeds. Certain bulls produce the daughters which have higher incidence of cystic ovaries.

- **Age :** Incidence is higher in that lactation in which milk yield is in peak. Therefore, ovarian cyst is *uncommon in first lactation.*

- **Nutrition :** Feeding of high protein diets causes higher incidence of the disease.

- **Season :** Incidence is more in winter than other seasons.

- **Stress :** Ketosis, dystocia, twin births, RFM, milk fever etc. cause stress. Due to stress, ACTH is released which causes LH suppression.

- **Postpartum uterine infections :** Endotoxin produced by micro-organisms in the uterus may trigger the $PGF_2 \alpha$ release, which in turn stimulates the secretion of cortisol. The elevated cortisol level suppresses the preovulatory release of LH and leads to the development of cyst.

Classification :

Ovarian cysts have been classified into two parts.

- **Anovulatory cyst or pathogenic ovarian cyst** eg. Follicular cysts and luteal cyst.

- **Ovulatory cyst or nonpathogenic ovarian cyst** eg. cystic corpora lutea.

    Follicular cysts : *are anovulatory follicles that persist on the ovary for 10 days or more, have a diameter greater than 2.5 cm. and are usually characterized by nymphomania.*

    Luteal cyst *is anovulatory follicle over 2.5 cm. in diameter that is partially luteinized and persists for a prolonged period and is usually characterized by anoestrus.*

    Cystic corpora lutea : are nonpathogenic ovarian cysts which arise following ovulation and are defined as corpora lutea that contain a fluid filled central cavity of variable size. Cystic corpora lutea are capable of normal progesterone synthesis and do not alter the length of the oestrous cycle.

Differences between follicular cyst and Luteal cyst :

Follicular cyst	Luteal cyst
1. Multiple on one or both ovaries.	1. Usually single in one ovary.
2. Thin walled as they do not get luteinized.	2. Thick walled due to partial luteinization.
3. Tense and distended, give fluctuating fluid-filled feeling.	3. Soft but luteinized tissue, gives little hard feeling.
4. More than 2.5 cm. in diameter	4. About 2.5 cm. or slightly more.
5. Persist for 10 days or more.	5. Persist for a month or longer.
6. Easy to rupture.	6. Difficult to rupture.
7. Fluid inside the cyst is pale yellow or straw-coloured.	7. Fluid is usually amber or dark yellow or brown in colour.
8. Characterized by nymphomaniac symptoms.	8. Characterized by anoestrus.

Clinical signs of follicular cysts :

- Nymphomania i.e. displaying excessive and prolonged signs of oestrus, and a short interval between two successive oestruses.
- Excess swelling of vulva.
- Frequent and copious vaginal discharge than normal.
- Nervous, restless and bellowing frequently than normal.
- Attempt to ride other cows and will stand to be mounted by other cows.
- Sexually aggressive as a bull, so the affected cow is often spoken "buller".
- Relaxation of sacro-sciatic ligament.
- Sometimes *vaginal prolapse* when the cow sits down.
- *The mucus is tougher and more opaque than the mucus of oestrum.*

CLINICAL POINTER

The vaginal discharge is copious and opaque or whitish-grey in colour in this disease. Therefore, clinician may confuse with mucopurulent discharge. But when it is seen under microscope, there are usually no leucocytes in the mucus.

- External os of the cervix is usually large, dilated and relaxed.
- Uterus is large, oedematous and flaccid.
- In long standing cases of nymphomania, the relaxation of pelvic ligaments cause tipping of the pelvis and elevation of tail-head. This elevated tail head is called **sterility hump.**

CLINICAL POINTER
The sterility humps, in many cases persist after recovery of the disease because ligaments fail to regain their tone even after recovery. Therefore, a clinician should not be confused with sterility hump and presence of follicular cysts.

- **Hydrometra or mucometra is also found in long standing cases of follicular cysts.**

CLINICAL POINTER
The development of hydrometra or mucometra in the case of cystic ovaries results in cessation of heat and the owner believes that his/her cow is pregnant but after 6 to 8 months, the normal signs of pregnancy do not develop. Rectal examination reveals mucometra and cystic ovaries. Therefore, a clinician should be cautious during examination of cystic ovaries.

- **In few cases, cystic dilatation of the endometrial glands is so marked that the endometrium developed as *swiss-cheese appearance on histological section.***

INTERESTING FACT
It was previously believed that over-production of oestrogen is only responsible for nymphomaniac behaviours, but recent studies indicate that cows with follicular cysts, have blood oestrogen concentrations not much elevated than those in normal cows. Likewise testosterone concentration in cows with follicular cysts and nymphomania have no difference from the normal cows and cannot be correlated with the intensity of nymphomaniacal behaviour. Therefore, it may be concluded that it is not possible to correlate the concentrations of oestrogen, testosterone or progesterone in cows with cystic ovaries with their behavioural signs probably because both progesterone and testosterone modulate and potentiate the effects of oestrogen in the development of oestrous behaviour.

Clinical signs of luteal cyst :

- Cessation of cyclic activity i.e. *anoestrus.*
- Some of the long-standing cases of luteal cysts develop a masculine body and attempt to mount the other cows but *unlike the nymphomaniacal cow, they will not stand when being mounted by other cows.* This condition is called *virilism.*

INTERESTING FACT
Follicular cysts undergo cyclic changes i.e. they alternately grow and regress but fail to ovulate. Luteal cyst also fail to ovulate but persist for a prolonged period.

Diagnosis :

- The diagnosis of ovarian cyst is usually based on history, symptoms and on a clinical examination.

- A normal preovulatory follicle may approach 2.5 cm. in diameter. Its palpable characteristics of being a thin-walled, fluid-filled, smooth structure raised above the surface of the ovary may be confused with follicular cyst. For this, see the changes in uterus palpation and its symptoms.

- Corpus luteum in various stages of development and regression may be confused with ovarian cysts. During the first 5 to 7 days of the oestrous cycle, the developing corpus haemorrhagicum may be smooth and soft but after then, the corpus luteum becomes more liver like in consistency and be easily differentiated from an ovarian cyst.

- The accuracy of diagnosis can be markedly improved by use of transrectal ultrasound imaging.

- A follicular cyst may be associated with anoestrus, or with short oestrous cycles or with nymphomania. A follicular cyst causing nymphomania is not difficult to diagnose by a clinician, but distinguishing between follicular and luteal cyst in a cow which is in anoestrus, is more difficult.

Treatment of follicular cysts :

Various approaches to the treatment of ovarian cysts have been used since the disease was first described in 1831.

1. **Manual rupture :** Manual rupture of cystic structures by palpation per rectum. Ovarian haemorrhages and adhesions may follow manual rupture, which could further cause infertility. Therefore, manual rupture should be discouraged.

2. **Gonadotrophin-releasing hormone (GnRH) :** After treatment with GnRH analogue (Buserelin), most of the cows that respond come in oestrus 18 to 23 days after treatment. Receptal (Buserelin) – 5 ml I/M.

INTERESTING FACTS
• Previously it was thought that GnRH or hCG administration causes luteinization of the cyst by increasing the LH secretion. Recent studies indicate that GnRH has little direct effect upon the cyst itself but, instead, it causes ovulation of new follicles. These follicles develop into corpora lutea. Thus whether GnRH induces luteinization of the cyst or the formation of new corpora lutea, the result is an increase in progesterone concentration usually within 10 days of treatment. Elevated progesterone concentration causes a negative feedback resulting into decline in LH secretion leading to decreased oestradiol- 17 β concentrations. This is considered to be the most important factor in restoring normal cyclical activity.
• Some cows that failed to respond to GnRH treatment or with recurrent cyst, can be given second dose of GnRH.
• The cause of failure in response of GnRH treatment may be due to the degeneration of the cyst wall which prevents the thecal cells from responding to LH stimulation or occurrence of recurrent cyst.

3. **Administration of hCG :**

Chorulon (hCG) - 3000-5000 IU- I/V

Cows that respond to the treatment develop a normal oestrous cycle within 20 to 30 days after treatment. A second or third treatment may be required in few cases. Cases of ovarian cyst are not usually retreated until at least 3 to 4 weeks have elapsed and unless signs of nymphomania persist.

GnRH Versus hCG
GnRH is a small molecule and thus, has an advantage over hCG in the treatment of ovarian cyst since it is less likely to stimulate an immune response like hCG that reduces the effectiveness of subsequent treatment. Anaphylaxis following GnRH treatment has not been reported like hCG.

4. **Sequential GnRH and PGF$_2$α treatment :** Ovarian cysts that luteinize in response to GnRH administration undergo regression similar to that of normal corpora lutea. The luteolytic activity of PGF$_2$α reduces interval from the treatment with GnRH to the first oestrus (18 to 23 days). PGF$_2$α should be given on 9th days, after GnRH treatment.

0 day	-	Receptal	5 ml I/M
9th day	-	Lutalyse	5 ml I/M
11st day	-	Double A.I.	

INTERESTING FACT
Fertility in cows given PGF$_2\alpha$ 9 days after GnRH is similar or lower than the cows given only GnRH. Thus this regime reduces the time interval only.

5. Administration of progesterone :

50 to 100 mg progesterone (Duraprogen) I/M for 14 days or a single dose of 750 to 1000 mg repository progesterone is used for the treatment of follicular cyst.

CLINICAL POINTER
Conception rate in cows that respond to progesterone treatment are approximately 50 percent which is lower than that reported following treatment with hCG and GnRH.

Treatment of luteal cyst :

- PGF$_2\alpha$ analogue   - Lutalyse 5 ml – I/M

Prevention :

1. **Selective breeding :** The use of only such bulls whose daughters have shown low incidence of ovarian cyst.

2. GnRH treatment on days 12 to 14 post-partum reduces the incidence of ovarian cysts.

OBSERVATIONS :

Date ....

- Case No. ....
- Age of animal ....
- Species..
- Breed ....
- Date of parturition ....
- Nature of parturition ....
- Interval of oestrus cycle ....
- Symptoms of heat ....

- Nature of vaginal discharge ....
- Duration of heat ....
- Finding of *per rectal* examination
  Ovary   Left .... Right ....
  Uterine horn   Left............. Right ....
- Fern pattern ....
- White side test ....

Diagnosis ....

Treatment

    Rx

        1.   ....

        2.   ....

        3.   ....

        4.   ....

EXERCISE :

1. Why incidence of ovarian cyst is higher in between 4 to 6 years of age ?

Ans.

2. Why incidence of ovarian cyst is lower in first lactation ?

Ans.

3. Why does ovulation not occur in follicular or ovarian cyst ?

Ans.

4. What is the predominant symptoms of follicular cyst ?

Ans.

5. What do you mean by the term 'buller'?

Ans.

6. What indicates 'sterility hump' in a cow ?

Ans.

7. What is 'adrenal virilism' ?

Ans.

8. What is the reason behind occurrence of hydrometra or mucometra in long standing cases of ovarian cyst ?

Ans.

9.   What do you understand by the term 'swiss-cheese appearance'?
Ans.

10. Manual rupture of the ovarian cyst is contraindicated. Why ?
Ans.

11. GnRH treatment is better than hCG treatment. Give reason.
Ans.

12. What will you do for prevention of ovarian cyst ?
Ans.

❊ ❊ ❊ ❊ ❊

It is bad plan that admits no modification.

- Syrus

Chapter 31

Diagnosis and Therapeutic Management of Repeat Breeder Cows

Definition :

A cow/ buffalo which has normal or nearly normal oestrous cycle and oestrus period and has been bred or artificially inseminated three or more times continuously to a fertile bull or with semen of fertile bull yet failed to conceive, is called a repeat breeder.

Causes :

Failure of fertilization and **early embryonic death** are two main reasons responsible for repeat breeding syndrome.

- Anovulatory heat
- Delayed ovulation
- Early embryonic death
- Failure of nidation of fertilized ovum
- Deficiency of energy
- Deficiency of progesterone
- Excess of oestrogen
- First degree endometritis
- Aged sperm and ovum
- Poor hygiene at the time of calving and A.I.
- Poor management and handling of frozen semen
- High ambient temperature and humidity
- Urovagina
- Pneumovagina
- Malnutrition

Diagnosis and treatment :

1. **Anovulatory heat and delayed ovulation :**
    *   Examine the ovaries on the day of oestrus and record the location of follicle.
    *   Examine the animal again first day and second day, considering the day of oestrus as zero to know whether the ovulation has occurred or not.
    *   If ovulation occurs, there will be a ovulatory depression on the ovary in place of mature Graafian follicle.
    *   If the animal ovulates second day or later on, it is a case of delayed ovulation.
    *   In case of delayed ovulation, a cow can be inseminated two or three times at 12 hours interval.
    *   Examine the ovaries on 9th or 10th day of oestrus for presence of corpus luteum. If corpus luteum is not present on the ovary, it is a case of anovulatory heat.

INTERESTING FACT
Record rectal temperature in the early morning (before the animal get up) on the day of heat and on the following two days. If the temperature falls by 1^0F, it indicates that ovulation has occured on that day and so do A.I. accordingly.

Treatment :

GnRH analogues or hCG at the time of insemination to promote ovulation.

Dose : Receptal 2.5 ml. I/M.

2. **Early embryonic death within 16 days after A.I.**

When embryonic death occurs within 16 days of the cycle i.e. before maternal recognition of pregnancy (MRP), then the cow comes in heat at normal oestrous cycle length (18-22 days).

Causes of embryonic death :
*   **External factors :**
    *   Stress like pain & long transportation etc.
    *   Malnutrition
    *   Season and climate like summer

- **Maternal factors**
  - Progesterone deficiency
  - Uterine infection
- **Embryonic factors like chromosomal abnormalities**
- **Genetic factors**

Treatment :

- If early embryonic death occurs due to genetic cause, change of bull may help to overcome this defect.
- When early embryonic death occurs due to external or environmental factors, proper management may help to overcome this defect.
- Subclinical uterine infections also cause early embryonic death. For this, intrauterine or systemic antibiotic therapy is indicated. Most common treatment in practice is to do pre- AI antibiotic treatment or post-AI antibiotic treatment: For this, 10 lakh IU penicillin or 1gm. streptopenicillin should be dissolved in 20-30 ml. of distilled water. Few veterinarians use 250 mg. ampicillin & cloxacillin or 200 mg (5 ml) gentamicin in 30 ml. distilled water. Pre AI treatment should be given 5 to 6 hours before AI while post AI treatment should be given 3 to 6 hours after AI. Parenteral antibiotics (preferably strepto penicillin 2.5 gm.) should be given on day 4 and on day 10 because zygote comes to uterus on day 4 and zona hatching and nidation of embryo occur around the day 10; so that the antibiotics enters into the uterine fluid around these periods and controls the infection.
- Embryonic mortality can occur due to heat stress, **so the inseminated cow/ buffalo should be kept in a cool place or in sheds for 15 days after insemination.** Adequate access to water and cooling with water is also highly effective.

Progesterone deficiency :

- Corpus luteum is the source of progesterone. If it is not completely formed or it is not functioning adequately, then insufficient progesterone causes pregnancy failure.
- Therefore, progesterone should be administered 3 to 5 days after insemination and continued for a variable period of 2 to 3 weeks which improves the conception rate in repeat breeder cows that have luteal deficiency.

- Administration of hCG (2000 I.U. IM or 1000 I.U. I/V) 5 days after oestrus induces ovulation of the dominant follicle of first wave and formation of an accessory corpus luteum which increase the plasma progesterone level. In this way, it reduces the incidence of embryonic mortality. It gives better result than progesterone administration.

- Administration of GnRH analogue (Buserelin 10 μg. or 2.5 ml) on day 11 after insemination, reduces the embryonic mortality. It is believed that the main effect of GnRH is not luteotrophic like hCG but it reduces the oestradiol concentration resulting in a decline in $PGF_2\alpha$ release during critical period of early pregnancy. This provides the embryo with more time to produce **bovine trophoblastic protein or interferon tau.**

3. **Deficiency of oxytocin :**

   The lack of tonicity of uterus in an oestrous animal may be due to deficiency of oxytocin. **These animals may pass large quantity of urine when examined per rectally.** 30-50 IU oxytocin should be injected intramuscularly after insemination.

4. **Poor management :**

- Animal should **not be excited 15 minutes prior to, during or 15 minutes after AI.** Excitation causes the release of adrenaline thereby lowering the action of oxytocin which is required for sperm transport.

- In cattle, the **clitoris should be massaged** gently two to three times after AI. This helps in sperm transport and ovulation.

- **Cold water should be poured on the back** of the animal after AI which causes abdominal muscles contraction and in turn of uterine muscles and thus, helps in sperm transport.

- Fifteen minutes rest is necessary after AI so that the sperm can reach the utero-tubal junction.

- The owner should be given advice to **examine the mucosa of vulvar lips** of the animal daily for **"next three days"** to notice any pus-flakes, which is an indication of first or second degree endometritis and such cases should be treated appropriately in the next cycle.

- **Proper thawing of frozen semen** and AI should be done within few minutes after thawing.

- **Proper insemination technique** should be followed to deposit the semen just after the anterior end of cervix or in the body of uterus otherwise it will cause trauma to the genital tract.

5. **Deficiency of energy :**

If deficiency of energy is suspected, 20% dextrose intravenous should be given 1 to 2 hours prior to AI.

Energy Deficiency
• Animal should be in **positive energy balance**. Under-feeding of energy can cause delayed ovulation, anovulatory condition and embryonic death. The concentrate feed must contain mineral mixture at 2% level.
• **Energy deficiency** affect the fertility in two ways. First through **GnRH system** and the second through **metabolic regulators of ovarian function.**
• FSH secretion is not only largely affected by nutrition but LH secretion is also affected in negatively energy balanced animal resulting delayed ovulation, anovulation or early embryonic death.
• Metabolic regulators: The circulating concentrations of glucose, insulin and insulin like growth factor 1 (IGF-1) are lower in cows that are in negative energy balance than in fully fed animals while concentration of **non-esterified fatty acids (NEFA) are higher** in negatively energy balanced animals. All of these alter the gonadotrophin secretion affecting follicle development. Some studies indicate that NEFA have direct toxic effect on follicles and oocytes.

Suggested line of treatment :

- On the day of oestrus, ciprofloxacin and tinidazole combination (C-Flox-Tz 30 ml.) should be given intrauterine for 3 to 5 days. Insemination should not be done in this cycle.
- In the next cycle, 500 ml. 20% dextrose (Intalyte or Rintose) should be given intravenoulsy two hours prior to insemination.
- Immediately after AI, 1500 IU hCG or 2.5 ml. receptal should be injected.
- Oxytocin 30 IU should be given intramuscularly if atonicity of uterus is suspected.
- After 5 days of insemination, 500 mg progesterone (2 ml, duraprogen) should be given intramuscularly and repeated again on day 10.

212

- Parenteral antibiotic (preferably Streptopenicillin) should be given on day 5 and on day 10.

Crude protein
• The high level of crude protein (CP) in the diet has an adverse effect on the conception rate. Feeding of high level of rumen degradable protein (RDP) leads, to an increase in circulating concentrations of **ammonia** and **urea**. In consequence, abnormally high concentrations of urea and ammonia reach to the uterus, where they may be **toxic to spermatozoa** or **adversely affect uterine function and reduces the embryo survival rate.** In addition, abnormally high circulating concentration of urea may also have an adverse effect on the **hypothalamic-pituitary axis.**
• 20% dietary CPDM (crude protein dry matter) increases incidence of RFM, dystocia and post partum metritis as compared to 13% level.
• Interestingly, small improvement occurs when **undegraded rumen protein (UDP)** is present in the diet by neutralising the effect of RDP.
• Soyabean meal, fish meal etc. have high proportion of undegradable protein while protein in silage and barley is highly degradable.
• **Therefore, it can be concluded that high level feeding of protein should be avoided for maintaining the fertility of cow.**

OBSERVATIONS :

Date..............................

- Case No. ....
- Age ....
- Species ....
- Breed ....
- Number of calving ....
- Date of last calving ....
- Date of first heat ....
- Number of services failed ....
- Interval of oestrous cycle ....
- Gynaecological findings ....

	Left	Right
Ovary	....	....
Fallopian tubes	....	....
Uterine horns	....	....

Vagina and vulva ....

- Other history, if any ....
- Report of antimicrobial sensitivity test ....
- **Treatment given**

   Rx

   1.   ....

   2.   ....

   3.   ....

   4.   ....

EXERCISE :

1. Why progesterone should not be administered within 3 days after insemination ?

Ans.

2. What is the role of hCG administration after 5 days of insemination ?

Ans.

3. What is the symptoms of deficiency of oxytocin at the time of AI ?

Ans.

4. Why the animal should not be excited 15 minutes prior, during or 15 minutes after AI. ?

Ans.

5. What is the effect of clitoris massage after AI ?

Ans.

6. What is the effect of pouring of cold water on the back of the animal after AI. ?

Ans.

7. Fifteen minutes rest is necessary after AI. Why ?

Ans.

8. Why one should observe the vulvar lips for next three days after AI ?

Ans.

9. What is the effect of NEFA ?

Ans.

10. What is the effect of high level of feeding high level of rumen degradable protein ?

Ans.

Happiness springs from intense activity in congenial surroundings.

– Harold Nicholson.

Chapter 32

Principles of Antimicrobials Therapy

OBJECTIVES :

- To know the efficacy of antimicrobials in the treatment of uterine infections.
- To know the mode of action of antimicrobials on microbes.
- Selection of appropriate antimicrobial in different pathological conditions of uterus.

Criteria for an ideal intrauterine antimicrobials :

1. It should be broad spectrum.
2. It should be effective against both aerobic and anaerobic bacteria. Because uterine environment is mainly anaerobic so anaerobic bacteria flourish more than aerobic bacteria.
3. It should penetrate all the layers of uterus like endometrium, muscles and serosa.
4. It should not inhibit **natural defence mechanism of uterus.**
5. It should not be irritant.
6. It should be easily available and economical.
7. It should be **weak acid** when only endometrium is infected, because these drugs ionize more in uterine lumen than plasma. So at equilibrium, more concentration of drug will be found in uterine lumen.
8. It should be **weak base** when sub-endometrial layer is infected because weak base drugs more ionize in plasma i.e. more absorption of drugs occurs through uterine layers.
9. It should be effective **even in presence of pus in uterine** lumen.

Parenteral route versus intrauterine route :

Parenteral administration :

- Parenteral administration results in better distribution of drug in the whole tubular genital tract and to the ovaries than intrauterine administration.
- Foetal membranes and abnormal exudates cannot mechanically influence the distribution of drugs through parenteral administration than intrauterine route.
- Parenteral administration reduces the risk of damage to the endometrium in comparison to intrauterine route.
- Repeated treatment can be carried out relatively simply and without introduction of new infections in comparison to intrauterine route.

Intrauterine administration :

- Anaerobic condition of post-partum uterus prevents many antibiotics to act on micro-organisms because these require oxygen for their activity. eg. Aminoglycosides.
- **Pus, debris and blood in the uterus** reduce the effectiveness of many antimicrobials eg. **Sulphonamides, nitrofurans** and **aminoglycosides**. This results in unequal distribution of drug in subendometrial tissues, cervix, vagina, vulva, fallopian tubes and ovaries.
- It is not convenient method for repeated infusion.
- Infusion (drug) may damage the endometrium through trauma.
- Infusion may be expelled through the exudates.
- Further infection may be introduced to the uterus during intrauterine administration if hygiene is not maintained.

Selection of routes of administration
While deciding between systemic and intrauterine routes of administration, it is important to access the goal of therapy i.e. to produce therapeutic concentration of drug at the appropriate site in order to produce the desired result. If microbial growth is restricted to the lumen of uterus and endometrium then IU route would be better & economical. If invasion of micro-ogranisms have occurred into deeper layer of the uterine wall, then this would require the effective concentration of the antimicrobialin all regions of the genital tract. In this condition, systemic route should be preferred or both IU and systemic route.

Efficacy of uterine treatment with antimicrobial drugs :

Penicillin :

- Penicillins act by interfering with bacterial cell wall synthesis.
- The primary mechanism of resistance of some bacteria against penicillin is production of penicillinase enzyme which inhibits the action of penicillin.
- During early post partum period, many organisms in the uterus are capable of producing enzyme penicillinase that inactivates or degrades penicillins and cephalosporins. Therefore, during early postpartum period, penicillinase-sensitive antibiotics are not indicated for intrauterine therapy.
- Therefore, intrauterine administration of penicillin in the early and intermediate postpartum period is not likely to be effective.
- However, by 25 to 30 days post partum, only *C. pyogenes* and **gram-negative anaerobes remain in the uterus of most cows with metritis.** These bacteria are usually sensitive to intrauterine infusion of penicillin.
- One million (10 lakhs) units of intrauterine penicillin G procaine provide therapeutic levels for 30 hours in both the uterine lumen and the endometrium.
- A dose of 22,000 to 45,000 IU/kg is sufficient to combat most pathogens that are sensitive to penicillin because it provides serum levels higher than $1\mu g/ml$ for 6 to 12 hours in the wall of uterus.
- The average minimum inhibitory concentration (MIC) of penicillin for *C. pyogens* isolated from the bovine uterus is $1 \mu g/ml$.
- Clinical observation indicates that once daily dosage with penicillin is usually effective in the treatment of septic puerperal metritis even though serum levels may drop lower than $1\mu g/ml$ after 6 to 12 hours.
- Intramuscular administration of **10 mg estradiol benzoate significantly increases the absorption of penicillin** from the uterine lumen to uterine tissue.
- Systemic penicillin is acceptable because most of the bacteria **involved in invading the endometrium are Gram-positive** which are susceptible to penicillin.
- If penicillins are considered for intrauterine therapy, the semi-synthetic penicillins (ampicillin) are also preferred.

218

Oxytetracycline :

- Its mechanism of action is inhibition of protein synthesis at the level of the ribosome.

- Oxytetracycline is likely to be effective in the treatment of most of the mixed bacteria that exist in the **early postpartum uterus.**

- Therefore, oxytetracycline is the **antibiotic of choice for intrauterine therapy in the puerperal period if there is no septic infection.**

- Oxytetracycline concentration remains extremely **high in the lumen and endo metrium** after 24 hours of IU infusion, but **very low concentration in ovaries, oviducts, myometrium, serosa, cervix and vagina.**

- Oxytetracycline remain **active under anaerobic condition and also in presence of blood, pus and debris unlike other antibiotics, therefore, it is drug of choice for puerperal period.**

- Oxytetracycline at a dose rate of upto 22 mg/kg (recommended dose 11 mg/kg) provides MICs in uterine tissues as well as in lumen.

- Generally **injectable oxytetracycline** available in market containing **propylene glycol** as a vehicle or preservative should not be given by intrauterine route because it causes irritation to the endometrium.

- Therefore, **bolus form or powder form of oxytetracycline** should be used for intrauterine therapy.

Aminoglycosides :

- Gentamicin, kanamycin, streptomycin and neomycin are examples of amino glycosides that have been used in treatment of uterine infection.

- The mechanism of action of aminoglycosides is inhibition of protein synthesis at the level of the ribosome.

- The most important consideration in the use of aminoglycosides is that they enter the bacterial cell across a proton gradient generated by **oxidative phosphorylation, so they work well only under aerobic conditions.**

- In general, anaerobic bacteria are resistant to aminoglycosides because the drugs cannot enter the cells because of absence of oxidative phosphorylation in anaerobic bacteria.

219

- Therefore, aminoglycosides in uterus are ineffective in anaerobic environment of postpartum uterus.

Nitrofurazone :

- Activity of nitrofurazone is markedly inhibited by blood, pus and debris. All these factors are common to the postpartum uterus.
- One of the primary bovine uterine pathogens, ***C. pyogenes*** **is very resistant to nitrofurazone.**
- Nitrofurazone is irritating to the endometrium and causes shortened oestrous cycle when infused into the uterus of cows in diestrus.
- In a field trial evaluating treatment of pyometric cows, nitrofurazone infusion had a significant adverse effect on fertility.
- Consequently, recent studies indicate that nitrofurazone is contraindicated in the treatment of uterine infections.

Chloramphenicol :

Despite the fact that chloramphenicol is not FDA approved in most of the countries for use in food animals, it has received attention by practitioners because bacterial isolates from cows with post-partum uterine infection show resistance to the more commonly used antimicrobials. Sensitivity testing of cows with post partum reproductive problems revealed that chloramphenicol was the most effective antimicrobial tested.

Fluoroquinolones :

These are recently introduced which display a large volume of distribution, useful spectrum and unique mechanism of action. These can be usefully considered for parenteral treatment of metritis.

When faced with a challenge, look for a way, not a way out. – ***David Weatherford.***

Chapter 33

Diagnosis and Therapeutic Management of Post-partum Infections in Bovines

Relevances :
- Uterine infections are a major cause of economic loss to the cattle industry.
- Incidence of uterine infections are influenced by calving management, general sanitation, pathogenic organisms, endocrine factors, lactation, nutrition and other environmental stress factors.

Etiology, definition and classification of post-partum infections :

Etiology :
- The uterus is normally protected from bacterial contamination by the vulva, vestibular sphincter and cervix.
- During and immediately after parturition, these mechanical barriers are breached and the uterus is normally contaminated by a variety of pathogenic and nonpathogenic microorganisms.
- Most of these bacteria are only transient residents and are promptly eliminated by the uterine defence mechanism during the puerperium.
- In some cases, however, pathogens persist in the uterus and cause disease.
- The organism most commonly associated with uterine disease in cattle is *Actinomyces pyogenes*.
- The gram-negative anaerobes *Fusobacterium necrophorum* and *Bacteroides melaninogenicus* are frequently associated with *A. pyogenes*.
- *Bacteroides* decrease chemotaxis and inhibits phagocytosis by neutrophils allowing *A. pyogenes* to persist.

- A variety of other micro organisms are occasionally associated with uterine disease in cows and include *Coliforms, Pseudomonas aeruginosa, Staphylococci,* haemolytic *Streptococci* and others.
- *Clostridium* spp. occasionally infect the uterus and cause severe gangrenous metritis.
- Some of the organisms that transiently contaminate the uterus during the post-partum period produce penicillinase; this should be a considered during the selection of drugs and routes of administration.
- In cows with a normal puerperium, the uterus is nearly free of bacterial contamination by 4 weeks after calving.

Major groups of uterine bacteria :

- **Coliform bacteria**
  E. coli
  Proteus spp.
  Enterobactor spp.

- **Incidental bacteria :**
  Streptococci spp.
  Staphylocci spp.
  Pasteurella spp.
  Bacillus spp.

- **Corynebacteria :**
  C. pyogenes (now called *Actinomyces pyogenes*)

- **Gram negative anaerobic bacteria**
  Bacteroids spp.
  Fusobacterium spp.

- **Gram-positive anaerobic bacteria**
  Clostridium perfringes
  C. sporogenes
  Other Clostridium spp.

INTERESTING FACTS
• *C. pyogenes, Fusobacterium* and *Bacteroid* spp. act synergistically to enhance the diseases.
• *C. pyogenes* is the most significant pathogen of the intermediate and post ovulatory periods.
• Many types of bacteria intermittently inhabit the uterus in the post-partum period but most have little effect on fertility. However, they can give protection to the *C. pyogenes, Fusobacterium* and *Bacteroid* from the antibiotics because some of them secrete penicillinase which destroy the sensitive penicillins and cephalosporins.

Definitions :

- Definitions of uterine infections have considered character of uterine discharge, day postpartum, clinical findings and endocrine status.

- Unfortunately, clinicians and researchers have vaguely applied terms such as metritis and endometritis when describing uterine infections, which has contributed to confusion among veterinarians in the definition and economic impact of uterine infections.

- Therefore, specific definitions of related entities are presented as follows.

Postpartum period : It is defined as the period from parturition to complete uterine involution.

Metritis : Metritis is a result of severe inflammation involving all layers of the uterus (endometrial mucosa and submucosa, muscularis, and serosa).

Endometritis : Endometritis is characterized by inflammation of the endometrium extending no deeper than the stratum spongiosum.

Pyometra : Pyometra is characterized by accumulation of purulent exudates of variable amount within the endometrial cavity, persistence of a corpus luteum and suspension of the oestrous cycle.

Classification :

(a) Puerperal period :

It begins at the time of calving and continues until the pituitary gland becomes sensitive to GnRH at **7 to 14 days postpartum.**

(b) Intermediate period :

It begins with increased pituitary sensitivity to GnRH and continues until the **first post-partum ovulation.**

(c) Post ovulatory period :

It begins at the time of first ovulation and last until **involution is complete.** It is about **45 days** post-partum in normal cows.

Puerperal period :

● During the puerperal period, mixed populations of bacteria remain present in the uterus. Their numbers increase for several days, then start to decrease as involution progresses in normal cow.

● **RFM is a common problem of the early postpartum period** which increases the risk of uterine infections.

● Establishment of *C. pyogenes, Fusobacterium necrophorum* and *Bacterioides* **spp.** occur in this period, if condition is favourable. Eventually these get localize and cause chronic type of metritis in intermediate and postovulatory period.

● Coliform and incidental bacteria are decreased in number or eliminated from the uterus during the puerperal period especially in cows that develop more persistent infection with *C. pyogenes* and Gram-negative anaerobes.

● The coliform and incidental bacteria play no significant role in causing chronic metritis although in the early stages they may be associated with septic or toxic metritis.

● Life-threatening infection occur almost exclusively during this period like **septic puerperal metritis.**

● Many micro-organisms that cause septic puerperal metritis are susceptible to penicillin, so it is the antibiotic of choice for **systemic treatment** of the affected cows.

● In cows with **puerperal metritis without systemic involvement, local therapy** with **tetracycline alone** is usually adequate.

● **Oxytetracycline is the antibiotic of choice for intrauterine therapy in the puerperal period if there is no septic infection** (See the tetracyclines to know the reasons).

Intermediate period :

● In the intermediate period, bacterial populations are reduced in the uterus of normal cows.

- But in abnormal cow, uterine infection gets localized and causes **endometritis or metritis** and purulent discharge comes out when the cow lies down.
- Intrauterine infusion of **1-2 gm of tetracycline** in 20 to 40 ml. of sterile water or physiological saline solution is indicated because the uterus of many cows still contains mixed population of bacteria that may produce penicillinase. This therapy should be continued for a **minimum of 3 days.**

Post-ovulatory period :

- Most common diseases occuring in this period are **metritis** and **pyometra.**
- The bacteria that seems to be associated with the chronic metritis are *C. pyogenes* and **Gram-negative anaerobic bacteria** (*Fusobacterium necrophorum* and *Bacteroid* spp.)
- These bacteria stimulate exudation of large numbers of leukocytes resulting in purulent exudates.
- Since most metritis of this period is the result of penicillin-sensitive micro-organisms (*C. pyogenes* and **Gram-negative anaerobes**) because most of the other bacteria have been eliminated up to this period.
- So, penicillin is the antibiotic of choice for the treatment in the post-ovulatory period.
- Intrauterine infusion of **10 lakhs to 15 lakhs IU of penicillin** provides therapeutic levels in the lumen and entire wall of the uterus for a **minimum of 24 hours.**
- Normal healing of the endometrium after elimination of *C. pyogenes* requires about **a month. Therefore a cow should not be inseminated in next one or two oestrus periods.**
- Pyometra should be treated with oestrogen/ $PGF_2\alpha$ and antibiotics (Penicillin is the antibiotic of choice).

INTERESTING FACT
Inflammation of the oviduct, ovaries and ovarian bursa due to ascending infection from the uterus may be resolved and fertility may be restored in many cows but permanent functional impairment of oviductal epithelium may prevent successful fertilization and ova transport and the cow may become sterile.

Treatment :

Therapy for uterine infection has fallen into the broad categories of intrauterine therapy (antibiotics and antiseptic chemicals), systemic antibiotics and supportive therapy, and hormonal therapy.

Intrauterine Therapy :

- A variety of antibiotics and antiseptic chemicals have been infused into the uterus of cows in attempts to treat postpartum infections.

- The bovine uterus is an **anaerobic environment;** thus, antibiotics chosen for intrauterine use **must be active in the absence of oxygen.**

- In addition, most antibiotics and chemicals depress activity of uterine neutrophils and interfere with the uterine defence mechanism; therefore, the potential benefit of their use must be carefully weighed against their deleterious effects.

- Organisms that cause postpartum uterine infections usually are sensitive to penicillin, but bacterial contaminants during the first several weeks after calving produce penicillinase, which renders the drug ineffective if applied locally.

- By 30 days postpartum these organisms usually are eliminated, and intrauterine treatment with penicillin is more likely to be effective after that time.

- The daily intrauterine dose of penicillin recommended to reach the minimal inhibitory concentration (MIC) for *A. pyogenes* is 1×10^6IU.

- Oxytetracycline is commonly recommended for intrauterine therapy for post-partum infections. In a recent study, however, most isolates of *A. pyogenes* recovered from the uterus of cows were resistant to oxytetracycline and intrauterine treatment with large doses did not affect the frequency of *A. pyogenes* isolation.

- Furthermore, many preparations of oxytetracycline are **irritating and cause chemical endometritis.**

- **If oxytetracycline is selected for intrauterine therapy, doses of 4 to 6g/ day have been recommended in one study.**

- Intrauterine therapy with iodine solutions for the treatment of uterine infections is not recommended in all recent studies.

Systemic Antibiotics and Supportive Therapy :

- A variety of broad-spectrum antibiotics have been recommended for parenteral administration to cows with uterine infections.
- **Penicillin or one of its synthetic analogues is most commonly** recommended (20,000 to 30,000 IU/ kg *bid*).
- **Oxytetracycline probably is not a good choice for systemic administration because of difficulty in reaching the MIC required for** *A. pyogenes* **in the lumen of the uterus.**
- **Ceftiofur is a third-generation cephalosporin that has broad-** spectrum activity against both Gram-positive and Gram-negative bacteria has been founded useful in the treatment of metritis.
- Moreover, ceftiofur has been reported to reach **all layers of the uterus without violative residues in milk.**
- Subcutaneous or intramuscular administration of ceftiofur at a dose of 1 mg/kg in dairy cows after parturition result sufficient concentration of ceftiofur and its active metabolites in plasma, uterine tissues and lochial fluid that exceededingly reported MIC values for common pathogens involved in metritis.
- Ceftiofur administered at a dosage of **2.2 mg/kg. daily for 5 days** was efficacious in the treatment of metritis (rectal temperature >103.1^0 F with a foetid vaginal discharge).
- If dehydration complicates metritis, appropriate fluid therapy should be instituted and may be life-saving.
- Nonsteroidal anti-inflammatory drugs such as flunixin meglumine are used to combat toxaemia and improve appetite.
- Furthermore, cows with metritis may experience depressed appetite, affecting calcium and energy status. Consequently, **therapy with calcium and energy supplements may be warranted.**

Hormonal Therapy :

- A variety of hormones have been administered to cows in attempts to prevent or treat postpartum uterine infections.
- Oestrogen has been administered to initiate or strengthen myometrial contractions, but its use is **controversial.**
- **Contractions induced by oestrogen have been blamed for forcing the septic contents of the uterus not only through the cervix but also into the uterine tubes resulting in severe bilateral salpingitis.**

Uterine Defence Mechanism
• Normally, postpartum uterus has a heavy load of bacteria initially but these are eliminated by uterine defence mechanism in a normal cow. Phagocytosis of micro-organisms by neutrophils is an important bovine uterine defence mechanism. **This defence system is stimulated about 2 days after parturition by the invading micro-organisms.**
• Under pathological conditions, such as delivery of dead or weak calves, phagocytosis can be depressed for several days to several weeks.
• Trauma to the genital tract by removal of RFM and obstetrical procedures also depress phagocytosis.
• Possibly a number of antibiotics commonly placed in the uterus might also depress phagocytosis because of irritation.
• Uterine defence mechanism is stimulated by oestrogen and inhibited by progesterone.

- **Oxytocin causes contraction of the myometrium if the organ is dominated by oestrogen.**

- **Thus, oxytocin is expected to be effective in aiding uterine evacuation if administered within 48 to 72 hours after calving. Doses of 20 to 40 IU repeated every 3 to 6 hours are commonly used.**

- **Likewise cows affected with dystocia, RFM, or both and treated with $PGF_2\alpha$ in early post partum, followed by a second treatment of $PGF_2\alpha$ 14 days later, experienced a higher conception rate to first service than untreated cows experiencing a normal or abnormal parturition.**

- Prostaglandin is the drug of choice for therapy of pyometra. The evacuation of the uterus in 85% to 90% of treated cows occurs in 3 to 9 days after treatment but the endometrial lesions should be allowed 30 days to heal before A.I.

Prognosis :

- The prognosis for recovery from postpartum uterine infections varies with severity of the condition. Most cows with uncomplicated endometritis can be expected to recover.

- Metritis complicated by septicaemia may result in permanent impairment of fertility, decreased milk yield, laminitis, or in extreme cases, death of the patient despite aggressive treatment.

- Pyometra is rarely accompanied by abnormal clinical signs other than ansestrus in cows and rarely endangers the health or life of the animal. Most cows recover promptly from pyometra, if the condition is diagnosed and treated early in its course.

❊ ❊ ❊ ❊ ❊

We are taught to read but not trained to think. – *Dr. S. Radhakrishnan*

Chapter 34

Diagnosis and Therapeutic Management of Endometritis in Bovines

---

Definition :

"Inflammation of endometrium is called endometritis".

OR

"Inflammation of endometrium extending not deeper than the stratum spongiosum is called endometritis".

Predisposing factors :

- Retained foetal membranes
- Dystocia
- Multiple birth
- Abortion
- Induced calving
- Unsanitary calving condition

Etiology :

The principal micro-organisms associated with endometritis are :

(i) *Actinomyces pyogenes* (Previously called *Corynebacterium pyogens* Gram + ve)

(ii) *Fusobacterium necrophorum* (Gram-ve, anaerobic, non-spore forming).

(iii) *Bacteroid species* (Gram – ve, anaerobic, non-spore forming).

Physio-pathology of endometritis, chronic metritis and pyometra

Bacteria remain present in the uterus of 90 percent of dairy cows during the first 10 days post-partum. The composition of uterine flora in the post-partum cow has been found to **fluctuate constantly** throughout the first 7 weeks after calving as a result of **spontaneous contamination, clearance** and **re-contamination.** Leucocytes infiltration and phagocytosis eliminate invading organisms from the normal uterus. Phagocytosis of micro-organisms by neutrophils is important in the **bovine uterine defence system.** This defence system is stimulated about 2 days post-partum by the invading micro-organisms. Under pathological conditions, such as delivery of dead or weak calves, RFM, abortion etc. phagocytic activity remain depressed for several days to several weeks. Trauma to the genital tract also depresses phagocytosis.

During the puerperal period, mixed population of bacteria remain present in the uterus. Their numbers increase for several days and then decrease as involution progresses. If condition is favourable, *C. pyogenes, Fusobacterium necrophorum* and *Bacteroides* spp. become establish in the uterus. **Coliforms** and **incidental bacteria** get decreased in number or eliminated from the uterus during the puerperal period.

During the intermediate period (from pituitary sensitivity to the first postpartum ovulation), most of the pathogenic bacteria are reduced or eliminated in normal cows. Uterine infections that persist are referred to as **metritis or endometritis** and usually **signaled by a purulent vulvar discharge.**

Diseases occuring in the postovulatory period include **chronic metritis, endometritis** and **pyometra.** The bacteria that seem to be associated with more severe infertility are *C. pyogenes, Fusobacterium necrophorum* and *Bacteroides* spp. These bacteria stimulate exudation of large number of leucocytes, resulting in purulent exudates. If ovulation occurs before the uterus has expelled all the exudates and debris, the corpus luteum thatdevelops may be retained, the purulent exudates may be increased in volume, the oestrous cycle may be interrupted and pyometra may be **perpetuated.**

INTERESTING FACT

Within the uterus *A. pyogenes, Fusobacterium* and *Bacteroid* spp. act synergistically to enhance disease. *Fusobacterium necrophorum* produces a leucocidal endotoxin which intereferes with the host's ability to eliminates *A. pyogens*. Similarly *Bacteroid* spp. also produces substances that interferes with the phagocytosis and killing of the bacteria. These synergistic activities allow the establishment of *A. pyogenes* infections in the uterus. Duration of *A. pyogenes* infection determines degree of damage of endometrium.

Thus, *A. pyogenes* is responsible for the disease and the rest two bacteria (*act like body-guards*) give protection to it from uterine defence mechanism.

Clinical signs :

- White or whitish-yellow mucopurulent vaginal discharge comes out when a diseased cow sit down.
- Copious mucopurulent discharge at the time of oestrus.
- No signs of systemic illness like septic puerperal metritis.
- Repeat breeding and failure of conception are the most common symptoms of endometritis.

Classification :

(i) **Clinical endometritis :** When the uterine discharge is thrown by the animal, is mucopurulent, it is called clinical endmetritis.

(ii) **Subclinical endometritis :** When the uterine discharge is thrown by the animal is **almost clear,** but give positive reaction to **white side test,** this condition is called subclinical endometritis.

Degree of endometritis :

(i) **First degree :**

- The oestrous cycle is normal.
- Vaginal discharge is clear.
- Vaginal discharge remains clear even after squeezing from the tip to base of each horn (milking out of uterus).
- **On the 3ʳᵈ or 4ᵗʰ day of A.I., flakes of pus may be observed intravaginally or within vulvar lips.**

Diagnosis :
- White side test.
- When mucus discharge is examined under the microscope using a low power lens without staining, more number of WBC are seen as small dots, along with superficial epithelial cells (irregular contour cells). Under high power, more than 8 number of WBCs are seen per field.

(ii) Second degree :
- The oestrous cycle may be either normal or prolonged.
- Vaginal discharge is clear.
- **But on milking out of uterus, the discharge becomes cloudy or dirty.**
- The genital tract is slightly thick and heavy.

Diagnosis :
- White side test.
- Microscopic examination of the vaginal discharge.

(iii) Third degree :
- The oestrous cycle may be prolonged.
- **Discharge is mucopurulent** especially during oestrus.
- **The genital tract is felt distinctly thick and enlarged.**

Treatment :

Therapeutic approach of endometritis is based on :

Increased contraction of uterus to expel the mucopurulent content.

Stimulation of uterine defence mechanism.

Overcome the uterine infection.

Restoration of damaged endometrium.

(1) Antimicrobial therapy :

Intrauterine route : Most metritis or endometritis of the **late post partum period** is due to penicillin-sensitive *A. pyogens* and Gram-negative anaerobes because other bacteria have been eliminated by that time. **Therefore, penicillin is the antibiotic of choice fortreatment.** Intrauterine infusion of 10 lakhs to 15 lakhs IU of penicillin provides therapeutic levels in the lumen and entire wall of the uterus for a minimum of 24 hours.

CLINICAL POINTER

Since normal healing of the endometrium following elimination of *A. pyogenes* requires about a month therefore early post-treatment insemination fails.

- Aminoglycosides (Gentamicin) are not effective in the **predominantly anaerobic environment of the uterus.**
- Sulphonamides are ineffective because of **presence of pus.**
- Nitrofurazone (furea) **is irritant and has adverse effect on fertility. Also** *A. pyogens* **is very resistant to nitrofurazone.**
- Oxytetracycline treatment is effective in most of the **mixed bacterial infection that exists in the early post-partum uterus.** However, the action of locally administered **tetracyclines are limited primarily to the uterine lumen and the endometrium. Therefore, intrauterine therapy of oxytetracycline should be given when only the endometrium is infected at a dosage of 2 gm daily for 3 to 5 days.**

Parenteral administration :

- **Penicillins** (fortified procain penicillin injection 40 lakhs IU).

  Dose : 8000-10,000 IU per kg. body weight at 24 hours intervals for 3-5 days deep IM route.
- **Oxytetracycline :** A dose rate **upto 22 mg/kg IM or IV** provides effective MICs in the lumen and uterine tissues.

(2) Hormonal therapy :

(i) **Oestradiol valerate** – Dose 3 to 10 mg. I/M. This treatment can be repeated at an **interval of 7 days** if required.

(ii) **Oxytocin :** Administer low dose (10 to 20 IU) of oxytocin within 4 to 6 hours of the oestrogen injection.

These hormones increase the uterine tone and blood flow to the uterus. In this way, they increase the uterine defence mechanism and also help in evacuation of pus.

CLINICAL POINTER

Higher dose of oestrogen can cause severe inhibition of pituitary functions, **which affects the folliculogenesis resulting in cystic ovaries. Therefore, a lower dose of (3mg /500kg. b.w.) oestrogen is sufficient and safe for the treatment of chronic endometritis.**

(iii) **PGF$_2\alpha$ analogues :** When corpus luteum is present, PGF$_2\alpha$ is the most successful treatment both in terms of cure rate and calving to conception interval. Lutalyse 5 ml. I/M. or Vetmate 2ml. I/M.

(3) Supportive therapy :

Levamisole @ 2.5 mg/kg b.w. i.e. 10-15 ml. S/C can be given as an immunostimulant, one injection per weeks for two weeks.

Mineral mixture containing Vit. A, D & E helps in regeneration of damaged endometrium and enhances immunity and tone of the uterine muscles.

OBSERVATIONS :

Date ....

- Case No. ....
- Species ....
- Breed ....
- Age ....
- Date of parturition ....
- Nature of parturition   *Eutocia/Dystocia*
- Temperature ....^{0}F.
- Pulse rate ....$/$min.
- Respiration......................$/$min.
- Feed intake   *Normal/Less than normal/Nil*
- Water intake   *Normal/Less than normal/Nil.*
- Vaginal discharge ....
- Per-rectal finding ....
- Result of white side test ....
- Result of microscopic examination of vaginal discharge ....
- Degree of endometritis ....
- Endometritis   *Clinical/Subclinical.*
- **Treatment**
  Rx.
  1.   ....
  2.   ....
  3.   ....
  4.   ....

EXERCISE :

1. How can *Fusobacterium necrophorum* and *Bacteroid* spp. act in enhancing the uterine disease ?

Ans.

2. How will you diagnose the subclinical endometritis ?

Ans.

3. What is the drug of choice for combating uterine endometrial infection during early post-partum period and why ?

Ans.

4. What is the drug of choice for combating endometritis during late post-partum period and why ?

Ans.

5. After how many days of treatment of endometritis, AI should be done and why ?

Ans.

6. What is the side effect of high dosage of oestrogen injection ?

Ans.

7. Why oxytocin is given after oestrogen administration in the treatment of endometritis ?

Ans.

✖ ✖ ✖ ✖ ✖

Words are the most powerful drug used by mankind.

Diagnosis and Therapeutic Management of Septic Puerperal Metritis

---

Puerperal metritis :

Metritis is the inflammation of the entire thickness of uterine wall (endometrium, myometrium and serosa). When it occurs just after parturition, it is called puerperal metritis.

Predisposing factors :
- Dystocia
- Twin births
- Retention of foetal membranes
- Prolonged traction and damage of birth canal
- Unsanitary calving condition

Under such conditions, the chances of invasion of the uterus and multiplication of large number of pathogenic bacteria get increased.

Etiology :
1. *Corynebacterium pyogenes* (Now, *Actinomyces pyogenes*) – **Most important bacteria.**
2. *Streptococci* (group C).
3. *Staphylococci* (haemolytic).
4. Coliform bacteria: *E. coli, Proteus* and *Enterabacter* spp.
5. Gram-negative anaebrobes (*Bacteriodes* & *fusobacterium* spp.)
6. Gram-positive anaerobes (*Clostridrium* spp.) rarely

These bacteria get colonised in the non-involuted uterus, some of which are producing toxins which are absorbed and cause severe symptoms.

Pathogenesis :
Failure of normal involution combined with retention of the foetal

membranes and infection of the uterus with a mixed bacterial flora resulting in acute metritis and severe toxaemia. There is diffuse necrosis and oedema of the mucosa and wall of the uterus. There is marked accumulation of foul-smelling fluid in the uterus, and thereby enlargement of the uterus. Absorption of toxins cause in severe toxaemia.

Symptoms :

- The septic puerperal metritis exclusively occurs during puerperal period i.e. within 2-4 days after parturition.
- Affected animals show both local and general symptoms.

General symptoms :

- Depression
- Anorexia
- **Hyperthermia followed by hypothermia**
- Tachycardia (96-120 beats/min)
- Respiration rate high (60-72 times/min, normal 15-20 times/min)
- Cool skin and extremities
- **Foul-smelling diarrhoea**
- Dehydration because the affected cow does not drink normally
- Anuria
- Congested mucosa with an increased capillary refill time
- Muscular weakness, leading to recumbency
- Marked drop in milk production
- Rumen contraction reduced or absent
- Septic shock and death

Localized symptoms :

- **Large quantities of foul-smelling, dark brown to red fluid** containing pieces of degenerating foetal membranes comes out from the uterus through the vagina.
- **Frequent straining.**

DIFFERENTIAL DIAGNOSIS
Puerperal metritis must be differentiated from **pneumonia**, traumatic reticulitis, left side displacement of the abomasum because their general symptoms are likely to match with the puerperal metritis and they also occur during puerperial period.

Treatment :

1) **Antimicrobial therapy** e.g., penicillins, I/M or IV for several days until recovery occurs.

2) **Non steroidal anti-inflammatory drugs :**

   Ketoprofen : Dose : 3 mg/ kg b.w. I/M or I/V at 24 hours interval.

   Trade name – Neoprofen 15 ml vial containing ketoprofen 100mg/ml.

   Meloxicam : Dose 0.5 mg/kg b.w. at 24 hours interval.

   Trade name -Melonex (Intas) 15 ml & 30 ml vial containining meloxicam 5 mg/ml.

(3) **Antihistamines** eg. Chlorpheniramine maleate and pheniramine maleate.

   Pheniramine maleate (Avil)

   Dose 5-10 ml. I/M

   Chlorpheniramine maleate (Codistin, Zeet etc.)

   Dose – 30-50mg (total dose) i.e. 3-5 ml I/M.

(4) **Glucocorticoid (Dexamethasone)** should be used in severe case to prevent septic shock.

   Dose – 10-30 mg (total dose) or 5 ml. I/M or I/V every 24 hours.

(5) **Fluid and electrolytes :-** The intravenous infusion of large quantities of fluids and electrolytes is essential in the management of septic puerperal metritis. Large volume of isotonic fluids have been standard practiced. Lactate Ringer's solution or a balanced electrolyte mixture must be given by IV infusion over several hours. Glucose should be included in the infusion fluids.

BENEFITS OF FLUID & ELECTROLYTE THERAPY
• Correction of peripheral vasoconstriction.
• Restoration of an acceptable pulse quality
• Return of urinary output.
• Restoration of cardiac out put.
• Dilution of toxins.

(6) If the cow is continually straining, **caudal epidural anaesthesia can be used;** gives temporary relief for 1-2 hours and sometimes it will break the cycle and stop the straining.

CLINICAL POINTER
The use of oestrogen is contraindicated in cases of acute puerperal metritis because oestrogens increase the contraction and blood flow in the uterus thereby increasing the absorption of bacterial toxins and thus, the case becomes more severe.

(7) **Remove the retained foetal membranes** by very gentle external traction, if possible otherwise leave it as it is.

CLINICAL POINTER
The hand should not be entered in the vagina and uterus to remove the placenta. Because the uterus in this condition is friable, it may result in severe damage and also predispose to the absorption of toxins and making the case more severe.

(8) **Intrauterine medication :** Intrauterine medication is **controversial** because in the acute puerperal metritis, it does not eliminate infection. Intrauterine infusion of oxytetracycline does not penetrate all the layers of the uterine wall. Penicillins through intrauterine route are also ineffective because in early postpartum period, there are mixed bacterial environment in the uterus. So penicillin-resistant organisms provide protection to penicillin-sensitive pathogens. Therefore, intrauterine administration of penicillin in the early and intermediate postpartum period is not likely to be effective. After the initial improvement like when temperature approaches normal, resumption of appetite and cessation of diarrhoea then, **intrauterine antibiotics should be started.**

Selection of antimicrobials :
Selection of antimicrobials for the treatment of acute puerperal metritis parenterally is very important. Most organisms that cause septic puerperal metritis are susceptible to penicillin, so it is the antibiotic of choice of systemic treatment of the affected cow.

(9) **Vitamin B-complex with liver extract :** intramuscular for three days.

Prognosis : The prognosis for subsequent fertility should always be guarded, because cows that have suffered a severe puerperal metritis very often develop lesions such as **ovario-bursal adhesions, uterine adhesions and occluded uterine tubes.**

OBSERVATIONS :

Date : ....

- Case No. ....
- Species ....
- Breed ....
- Age ....
- Date of parturition ....
- Time of parturition ....
- Nature of parturition   Eutocia/Dystocia
- Temperature ....°F
- Pulse rate ..../min.
- Respiration rate ..../min.
- Feed intake ....*Normal/Less than normal/complete anorexia.*
- Water intake .... *Normal/Less than normal/Nil.*
- Urination .... *Normal/Less than normal/Nil.*
- Ruminal movement .... *Normal/less than normal/Nil.*
- Rumination ....
- Vaginal discharge ....
- Placenta   *Retained/Removed normally/Removed manually*
- Straining   *Absent/Present*
- Diagnosis ....
- **Treatment** ....
  Rx
       1.
       2.
       3.
       4.

Results :

- Time of recovery ....
- Complications ....

EXERCISE :

1. Which is the most important predisposing factor for septic puerperal metritis?

Ans.

2. What is the drug of choice for the treatment of puerperal metritis and why ?

Ans.

3. Why fluid therepy is essential for the management of puerperal metritis ?

Ans.

4. Why oestrogen treatment is contraindicated for the treatment of acute puerperal metritis ?

Ans.

5. Why Vitamin B-complex with liver extract should be given during the treatment of puerperal metritis ?

Ans.

❈ ❈ ❈ ❈ ❈

The purpose of negative emotions is to help us survive and that of positive emoltions to help us succeed.

Chapter 36

Diagnosis and Therapeutic Management of Pyometra

Definition :

"Pyometra is accumulation of pus in the uterus

OR

" Pyometra is characterized by the accumulation of pus in the uterus and by a retained corpus luteum with failure of oestrus".

Predisposing factors :

Bovine pyometra is usually sequel or after-effect of abnormal parturition like abortion, pre-mature birth, twin births, dystocia, retained placenta, septic metritis or postpartum metritis. Under such conditions, the chances of invasion and multiplication of large numbers of pathogenic bacteria get increased inside the uterus.

Etiology : The most common infectious agents associated with pyometra are :

* *Corynebacterium pyogenes* or *Actinomyces pyogenes* (G+ve bacteria)
* *Fusobacterium necrophorum* (G-ve, anaerobes)
* *Bacteroides* **spp.** (G-ve, anaerobes)
* *Trichomonas foetus* (Protozoa)

Clinical Signs :

* In postpartum pyometra, the cervix does not remain too tight. So some of the pus escapes when the cow lies down, urinates or defaecates.
* Fail to show oestrum symptoms.
* On *per-rectal* examination :
    - Uterus remains enlarged on one side or both the sides.
    - . Uterine wall is thicker than what it is during pregnancy
    - Presence of corpus luteum

243

- Uterus has more 'doughy' (uterus is felt like soft balls of wheat-flour when fingers are pressed into)
- No caruncles
- No fremitus

Pathogenesis

Postpartum period is divided into three phases (details discussed in other chapter). During the **puerperal period**, mixed populations of bacteria remain present in the uterus. Their numbers remain increased for several days and then decrease as involution progresses. But if conditions are favourable, *C. pyogenes, Fusobacterium necrophorum* and *Bacteroides* spp. get established. In the **intermediate period** (up to the First postpartum ovulation), pathogenic bacteria are reduced or eliminated from the uterus of normal cows. Uterine infections that persist cause endometritis or metritis and are usually a signal for pyometra. In the **post-ovulatory period,** these bacteria (*C.pyogenes, Fusobacterium necrophorum* and *Bacteroides* **spp.** act synergistically) stimulate exudation of a large number of leucocytes resulting in pus formation. The corpus luteum of the first postpartum ovulation persists because chronic inflamed endometrium does not form $PGF_2\alpha$. The corpus luteum starts to secrete progesterone which favours the growth of micro-organisms and the cervix remains closed. In this way, pus gets gradually accumulated in the uterus.

Trichomonas foetus colonizes in the uterus. This particular protozoan species does not prevent fertilization but causes embryonic death at an early stage of gestation, sometimes embryonic death is followed by development of pyometra and persistence of corpus luteum.

Treatment :

1. Hormonal therapy :

(a) **Oestrogen and Oxytocin therapy :**
- Oestradiol valerate 3-10 mg. intramuscularly followed by Oxytocin 20 IU – 40 IU 24 hours later to sensitize the myometrium and dilate the cervix.
- Within 24 to 72 hours, most or all of the pus is usually expelled. If this has not occurred, second or third treatment with lower doses (2-5 mg) may be necessary at 2 to 3 days intervals.

(b) Oestrogen and glucocorticoid therapy :

The use of oestradiol valerate (10 mg or 1 ml. I/M) followed by dexamethasone (5 ml. I/M) have good result where oestrogen alone has failed.

(c) PGF$_2\alpha$ analogues :

- The best treatment is the use of PGF$_2\alpha$ analogues like lutalyse (5 ml I/M), Vetmate (2 ml I/M) etc. These cause regression of the corpus luteum, dilatation of the cervix and expulsion of pus within 5-7 days. Evacuation of the uterus is indicated by the signs of oestrus.

- The success of the treatment is indicated by the return of the uterus to normal condition, assessed by palpation within 7 to 10 days.

- The small percentage of animals that fail to completely evacuate of pus after the first treatment, 2nd injection may be repeated 8 to 12 days after the first.

- 40 to 70% conception rates following prostaglandin treatment are reported

2. Antimicrobial therapy :

- **Parenteral antibiotics** should be administered during the hormonal treatment because it prevents spread of infection to the oviducts due to contraction of uterus (preferably penicillin group).

- If an antibacterial drug is to be **infused into the uterine lumen** after expulsion of pus, **penicillin is the drug of choice** because after 25 to 30 days postpartum only *C.pyogenes* and Gram-negative anaerobes remain in the uterus of most of the cows with metritis or pyometra. These bacteria are usually sensitive to intrauterine infusion of penicillin (10 lakh IU).

- Other antibacterials such as tetracyclines or ampicillin are also useful.

Prognosis : The cases that have existed **only for 60 to 120 days**, recover and conceive more likely than the cases that have **existed for 120 days or longer**. In long standing cases the **endometrium gets destroyed**, the uterine wall undergoes fibrotic changes resulting in **permanent sterility**.

Oestrogens Vs PGF$_2$ α analogues

- The uterine contraction produced by **oestrogens** may spread the infection to the oviducts, ovaries and ovarian bursa resulting in sterility.
- The repeated use of oestrogens may also cause **cystic ovaries**.
- PGF$_2$α analogue injection causes luteolysis and follicular development, the level of progesterone decreases and the level of endogenous oestrogen increases. Thus, PGF$_2$α is safer than oestrogens.
- In one study it has been repated that **oestrogen increase** and **PGF$_2$α decrease days-open** in treated cows compared with controls.

INTERESTING FACTS

- Some veterinarians think that pyometra is the chronic mucopurulent discharge which is seen 2 to 3 weeks following calving due to postpartum metritis. In narrow sense, this may be correct because there is pus in the uterus but most of these cases come into heat, cycles remain regular and the pus is expelled within 30 to 60 days after parturition.
- True pyometra exists for 60 to 90 or more days after parturition with failure of oestrus and persistency of the corpus luteum.
- After treatment and expulsion of the pus from the uterus; the cow should not be bred for 1 to 2 normal oestrus cycles.

OBSERVATIONS :

Date ....

- Case No. ....
- Species ....
- Breed ....
- Age of animal ....
- Date of last service ....
- Stage of gestation ....
- Physical conditions ....
- Findings of *per-rectal* examination

....
....
- Diagnosis ....

- **Treatment given**

  Rx

  1. ....
  2. ....
  3. ....
  4. ....

EXERCISE :

1. Why massage method of evacuation of pus is not recommended?

Ans.

2. Corpus luteum persists in pyometra. Give reason.

Ans.

3. What are the most common organisms responsible for pyometra?

Ans.

4. What are the side-effects of oestrogen therapy in case of pyometra ?

Ans.

5. $PGF_2\alpha$ analogue is the best choice of treatment for pyometra. Give reason.

Ans.

❈ ❈ ❈ ❈ ❈

> *To be successful, you must accept all the challenges that come in your way. You can't just accept only the ones you like.*

Chapter 37

Diagnosis and Therapeutic Management of Retention of Placenta

Definition : *Retained foetal membranes (RFM) is defined as non-separation of the foetal membranes by 12 hours after calving (some authors extend this period to 24 hours).*

Primary retention of placenta : The RFM which results from a lack of detachment of cotyledons from the maternal caruncles is called primary retention of placenta.

Secondary retention of placenta : The RFM which results from mechanical difficulty in expelling already detached foetal membranes (eg. uterine atony), is called secondary retention of placenta.

Physiopathology of RFM
Normal expulsion of foetal membranes is a complex process involving mechanical, enzymatic and hormonal factors.   **Mechanical force :**   With the birth of the foetus, the blood vessels in the foetal placenta collapse and the villi (They are found on the surface of cotyledons) become small and shrunken. After the expulsion of the foetus, the uterus continues to contract strongly for 48 hours and less vigorously thereafter. This contraction is necessary to prevent haemorrhage and to aid in the expulsion of the foetal membranes. These peristaltic and contraction waves besides doing the above function, also reduce the amount of blood circulating in the endometrium. There is a decrease in blood supply to the endometrium that causes dilatation or relaxation of the caruncular crypts which plays a major role in the separation of the **villi of cotyledons and the crypts of caruncles.**

RFM is basically due to failure of the villi of the foetal cotyledons to detach from the crypts of the caruncle. Due to contraction of the uterine wall and reduced blood supply, the caruncles become round from their oval shape and smaller in size, and crypts dilate. The villi also become small and shrunken. In this way, detachment of the foetal cotyledons occur from the endometrial caruncles.

Enzymatic action : The defect in caruncle-cotyledon collagen breakdown is also the cause for retention of the foetal membranes. Normally cotyledons secrete collagenase enzyme which dissolves the collagen (adhesive factor), thus the cotyledons and caruncles get separated.

Etiology :

- Uterine inertia
- Abortion
- Multiple births
- Still-birth
- Advanced age of cow
- Caesarean delivery
- Dystocia
- Short gestation period plus low calf weight
- Summer calving
- Sex of calf (male)
- Hormonal imbalance
- Induced delivery ($PGF_2\alpha$, Dexamethasone)
- Vit. A deficiency
- Vit. E deficiency
- Excess iron
- Infection (eg. Brucella, moulds, Vibrio spp. etc.)
- Placentitis

Clinical signs :

Non infectious or low grade infection :
- Hanging of the placenta.
- No foetid smell from the placenta.
- Normal appetite.

- Normal pulse and temperature.
- Milk yield normal.
- Placenta is normal in colour, moist and glistening.

Severe infection and/or prolonged duration :
- Anorexia
- High fever
- High pulse rate
- Reduced milk yield
- Straining
- Foetid smell from placenta
- Discoloured and dry placenta

Treatment :

(1) **Oxytocin :** 75-100 IU intramuscularly if used immediately after calving, reduces the rate of RFM. If placenta is not removed even after this treatment, but it has beneficial effect at the time of manual removal of placenta because to some extent it loosens the attachment between the cotyledons and caruncles.

> Use of oxytocin is of questionable after 24 hours of calving because by this time, the response to oxytocin becomes poor. Unfortunately in cattle practice, generally veterinarian is not consulted until after 24 hours of retention of placenta because until then the farmer has hoped for a spontaneous expulsion.

(2) **Indigenous preparations :** Many indigenous preparations are available in the market for removal of retained placenta for example *Uterotone liquid, Uterifit, Involon* etc. One of these should be used for the expulsion of retained placenta as well as these assist in manual removal of placenta in the condition when normal expulsion is failed after this treatment.

Dose – Loading dose of 200 ml. on the first day followed by 100ml. for 3 consecutive days. Double the dose for animals weighing above 400 kg. After manual removal of placenta, one of these preparation is indicated because these help in increasing the tone of uterus, cleaning of uterus i.e. help in removal of remnants of placenta, tissue debris and pus. These also help in timely involution of the uterine horns.

(3) **Manual removal of retained placenta :** If normal expulsion of placenta fails even after the treatment with above mentioned

drugs, then the placenta should be removed manually (see procedure of manual removal).

(4) Intrauterine treatment : After manual removal of placenta, 2-4 boli of suitable intrauterine preparations should be kept in the uterine horns. Many intrauterine preparations are available in the market. These are *Furea, Lixen IU, C-flox-TZ, Steclin, Povidone iodine bolus, Cleanex etc.* One of these should be continued for 3 to 5 days in suspension form i.e. infuse the prepared solution in the uterus with the help of a catheter.

(5) Parenteral antibiotics : If there is any chance of active infection, then parenteral antibiotics should be given for 3-5 days. Strepto-penicillin or oxytetracycline has a good effect.

(6) Epidural anaesthesia, antihistamines, non-steroidal antinflammatory drugs (NSAIDS), antibiotics and liver extract injections are given before handling the case.

(7) When retained foetal membranes are associated with uterine atony caused by hypocalcaemia, oxytocin and calcium borogluconate give good results.

Procedure of manual removal :

- Give epidural anaesthesia (5-7 ml lignocaine).
- Grasp the hanging placenta in the right hand and **twist like a rope** so that the placenta can be more easily managed (see Fig. 37.1 and 37.2).
- Introduce the lubricated left hand into the uterus. The hand should be inside the uterus but outside the placenta i.e. between the uterus and placenta (see Fig. 37.1 & 37.2).
- Grasp the individual cotyledon and its caruncle between the thumb and fingers and the two structures (cotyledon and caruncle) should be gently separated by **rolling, pushing and squeezing motion.** This may be aided by traction with the other hand (right hand).
- Remove or separate the cotyledons from the caruncles first which are near to the cervical area, then from non-gravid horn and lastly from the gravid horn. During this operation, tension should be maintained on the hanging placenta.
- Sometimes, especially in exotic and large breeds of cow or earlier removal of placenta, the ovarian end or cranial end of gravid horn may be out of reach from the hand but traction on the

placenta sometimes pull the apex of the horn nearer and removal of cotyledons from this portion becomes possible.

- It is highly desirable to remove all the foetal membranes and not leave any remnant in the uterus as far as possible because they act as **foci of infection.**

POINTS TO REMEMBER
• The use of epidural anaesthesia controls straining and **defaecation** and makes gentle removal of placenta in a more hygienic manner.
• During manual removal of placenta, it is highly advisable to wear gloves. If gloves are not available, a good massage of castor oil or any antiseptic cream over the entire hand and arm is advised.
• The layman's practices of tying a weight on the placenta is not indicated because the weight causes the cow to strain and causes premature and incomplete breaking of placenta, leaving a part of it still in the uterus. This weight may also cause invagination of the uterine horn and prolapse of uterus may occur.
• **Manual removal of RFM is contraindicated if the cow has fever because uterine damage increases the risk of septicaemia and perimetritis.**

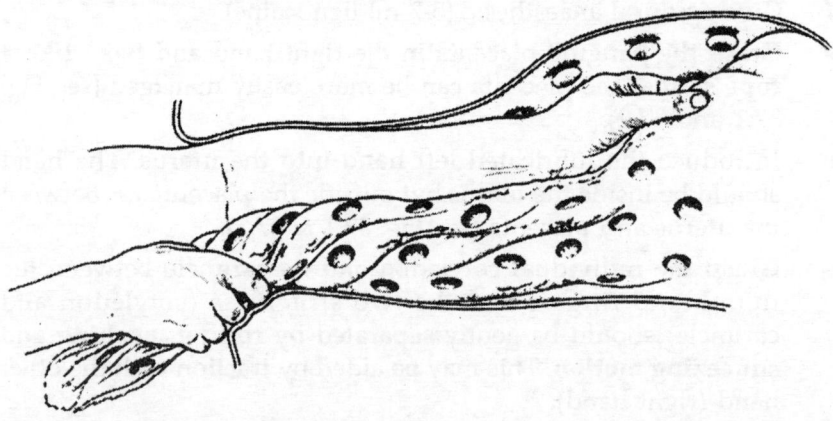

Fig. 37.1 : Manual removal of the placenta in a cow. The obstetrician grasps any protruding strand of placenta in one hand twists it into a 'rope' so that the placenta can be more easily managed. The other lubricated hands is introduced into the uterus. The hand should be inside the uterus but outside the placenta and the nearest attached caruncles and cotyledons should be searched for. (Courtesy of Jackson, P.G.G. 1995. Handbook of Veterinary Obstetrics. W.B. Saunders Company Limited).

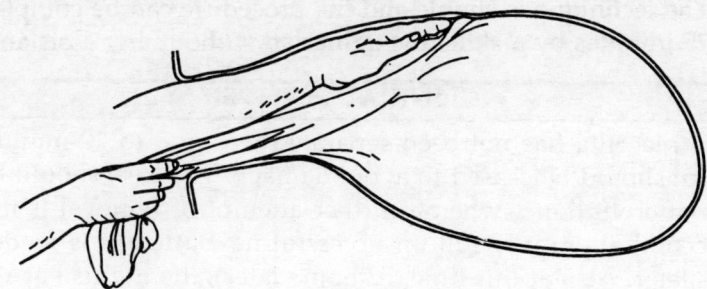

Fig. 37.2 : Manual removal of the placenta in a mare. (Courtesy of Jackson, P.G.G. 1995. Handbook of Veterinary Obstetrics. W.B. Saunders Company Limited).

Collagenase therapy :

- A new approach for the treatment of RFM is the injection of collagenase into the umbilical arteries.

- This approach may be superior to traditional treatments because it is specifically directed at correction of the lack of cotyledonary proteolysis.

- Bacterial collagenase from *Clostridium histolyticum* is used because it can degrade several types of collagen.

Technique :

- Locate the umbilical cord in RFM (recognized by two firm arteries and two veins of pencil-diameter that slip off from the fingers when palpated) by inserting one hand inside the vagina.

- Once the cord is located, second hand is also introduced into the vagina and the cord is retracted by alternating hands in the vagina.

- Once the umbilical cord is in the vulva, the arteries are clamped with Kelly's forceps.

- Inject collagenase solution (2 lakh units + 40 mg. calcium chloride + 40 mg sodium bicarbonate + 1 litre saline) rapidly.

- If antibiotic is desired, oxytetracycline (100 mg. total dose) can be added to 1 litre of collagenase solution.

Comments :

- Collagenase treatment is effective in 85% of affected cows within 36 hours.

- The treatment is safe and has no side-effect.

- The technique is simple and the procedure can be completed in 25 minutes by a skilled veterinarian without any assistant.

CLINICAL POINTER

If the placenta has not been separated within 5 to 20 minutes, the attempt should be ceased to avoid damage. The case should be seen again after 48 hours when a further attempt of removal is made. If the second attempt is still unsuccessful next attempt is made 48-72 hours later. Also at this time (72 hours later), the uterus has reduced in size so that the apex of the horn may be reached by hand. *Usually the cervix is still open sufficiently to allow passage of the hand and arm without resulting trauma.*

Effects of retained foetal membranes

- Reduced dry matter intake
- Low milk yield in that lactation
- Increased incidence of postpartum metritis, endometritis and pyometra.
- Increased time-period to first service
- Reduced conception rate/increased number of services per conception
- Increase days open
- Longer calving interval
- Predisposition of cows to other conditions such as left-displaced abomasum and laminitis

INTERESTING FACT

Manual removal is a superficially attractive method because it immediately removes the stinking (emitting an offensive smell) mass of decomposing tissue, thereby improving milking hygiene. However, there is increasingly controversial report that manual removal is detrimental to the cow.

Arguments in favour of manual removal :

1. It removes a major source of infection and putrefying protein.
2. It removes the unpleasant smell, which can taint the milk.
3. The cow may be less likely to develop systemic illness.
4. The cow may be less likely to have disturbed fertility later.
5. The cow may be less likely to suffer from reduced milk yield.

These points are not necessarily sufficient justification for manual removal of RFM, **point 2** is a benefit to the farmer rather than the cow and **points 3, 4 and 5** have been contradicted in many published trials. **Point 1 is** true, although there is little evidence that toxaemia occurs because the placenta has not been removed. Toxaemia can also occur after removal of the placenta.

Arguments against manual removal :

1. Just after calving, the cow is capable to eliminate a large amount of infected material and decomposing necrotic caruncles.

2. Intrauterine manual intervention should be avoided because it interferes with the natural defence mechanism by reducing phagocytosis for several days.

3. Manual removal of the membranes is never complete and numerous villi and remnants of placenta remain left attached.

4. Manual removal causes trauma and adds to the likelihood of local infection.

5. If the cow is ill, systemic treatment is sufficient to deal with the problem and manual removal may worsen the cow's condition.

6. Manual removal of the foetal membranes has a detrimental effect on fertility of the cow.

7. Manual removal has been found to prolong the interval from calving to the first functional corpus luteum by 20 days.

8. Attempts of removal during the first 48 hours after calving are unsuccessful because the placenta is too firmly attached and the apical part of the gravid horn is beyond the reach of the veterinarian.

OBSERVATIONS :

Date ....

- Case No. ....
- Species ....
- Breed ....
- Age ....
- History ....
- Date of parturition ....
- Time of parturition ....
- Sex of calf ....

- Parturition   *Normal/Abnormal*
- General condition :
  Temperature ....^{0}F
  Pulse rate ..../ min.
  Respiration rate ..../ min.
  Rumen motility ..../ min.
  Feed intake ....
  Water intake ....
  Micturation ....
  Straining ....
  Smell of placenta ....
  Colour of placenta ....
- Decision taken : ....
- **Treatment given**
  Rx

    1.
    2.
    3.
    4.

EXERCISE :

1. Manual removal of placenta is contraindicated in the febrile animals. Give reason.

Ans.

2. What are the benefits of epidural anaesthesia before manual removal of RFM ?

Ans.

3. Tying a weight on the hanging placenta is not advisable. Give reason.

Ans.

4. What is the role of contraction of uterus in separation of placenta ?

Ans.

5. What is the role of collagenase in separation of placenta ?

Ans.

6.   How will you locate the umbilical cord in RFM ?

Ans.

7.   The hanging portion of RFM should be twisted like a rope during manual removal. Why ?

Ans.

8.   Write the correct sequence of the areas of uterus from which RFM is separated ?

Ans.

9.   During the manual removal of RFM, gentle tension should be maintained on the hanging placenta. Give reason.

Ans.

❈   ❈   ❈   ❈   ❈

Confidence of success often induces real success. – Sigmund Freud.

Chapter 38

Diagnosis and Therapeutic Management of Vaginal Prolapse in Bovines

Vaginal prolapse :

- *"Protrusion of the whole or part of vagina through the vulva is called vaginal prolapse".*
- It occurs mostly in **late gestation (last 2 to 3 months of gestation).**

Pathogenesis :

If the pregnant animal is on the fodder containing oestrogenic property or large amount of oestrogen hormone is being secreted by the placenta, it cause relaxation of the pelvic ligaments, vulva and vulvar sphincter muscles. When the cow sits down, intra-abdominal pressure especially in late pregnancy is transferred to the flaccid pelvic structures which tend to force the relaxed and loosely attached vaginal floor and its wall through vulva.

Etiology :

1. Excess secretion of oestrogen hormone from the placenta.
2. Excess relaxation of pelvic ligaments.
3. Hypocalcaemia.
4. Excessive deposition of fat in the perivaginal connective tissue.
5. Oestrogenic feed (clover).
6. Inadequate exercise.
7. Bulky food (roughages).
8. Vaginal irritation.
9. Hereditary.

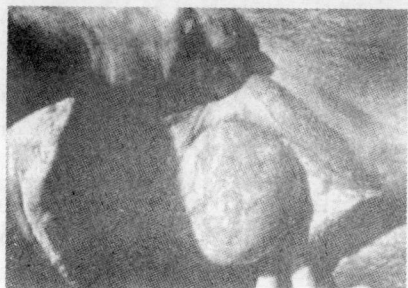

Fig. 38.1 : First-degree vaginal prolapse in a cow

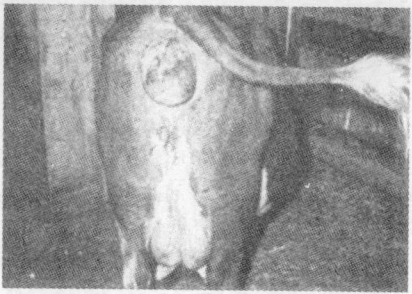

Fig. 38.2 : Second-degree vaginal prolapse in a cow

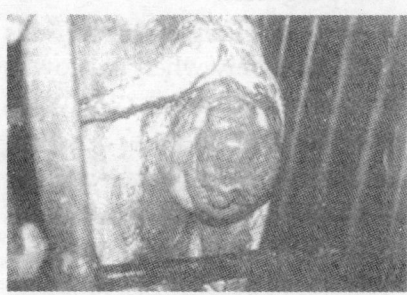

Fig. 38.3 : Third-degree vaginal prolapse. Note the cervical os dorsally and the oedamatous vaginal floor ventrally.

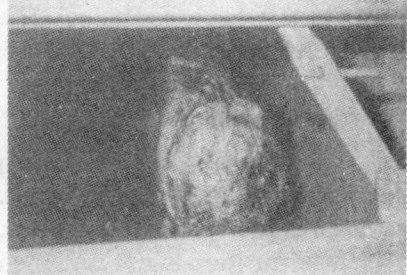

Fig. 38.4 : Fourth-degree vaginal prolapse. Note the fibrosis and necrosis

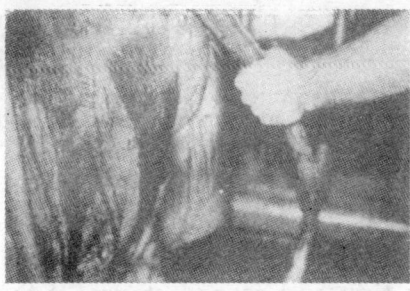

Fig. 38.5 : Primary cervical prolapse in an indigenous cow. (Courtesy of Wolfe, D.F. and Moll, H.D. 1999. Large Animal urogenital Surgery. Williams & Wilkins for All Figures of this Chapter).

CLINICAL POINTERS
• This condition is occasionally observed in cattle after parturition. At this time, it is often associated with cystic ovaries or other conditions characterized by excessive oestrogen production or severe straining.
• If prolapse of the vagina occurs during post partum period, the ovaries should always be examined for the presence of follicular cysts and if no cysts are present, then the vulva should be examined for injuries or inflammation.

Classification :

It is based on progression, severity and prognosis.

1. **First-degree prolapse : The floor of the vagina protrudes intermittently** through the vulva, usually only when the cow is lying down; but disappears when she stands up, is called first degree prolapse (Fig. 38.1).

   The vagina is irritated by exposure to sun, dust and faecal contamination. The vaginal mucosa is only congested with no damage to mucosa or infection. This stage usually go unnoticed. If parturition is not imminent (soon to happen), the continued vaginal irritation produces tenesmus, which leads to the next stage.

2. **Second-degree prolapse : The prolapse in which the floor of vagina is in continuous prolapse** even when the cow stands up is called second degree prolapse. If neglected the urinary bladder may be reverted into the prolapse, obstructing the urethra and interfering urination. (Fig. 38.2). Superficial erosion of vaginal mucosa may be found along with severe congestion, thickening and oedema of mucosa.

3. **Third-degree prolapse :** The prolapse in which both the cervix and almost the entire vagina remain protruded is called third-degree prolapse (Fig. 38.3). This may happen without progression through the first and second stages. If the cervical seal is disturbed, there is danger of septic abortion. The third–degree prolapse is also called **cervical prolapse.**

4. **Fourth – degree prolapse :** Second or third degree prolapse that has been exposed for a long period and necrosis and fibrosis has occurred, is called fourth degree prolapse (Fig. 38.4).

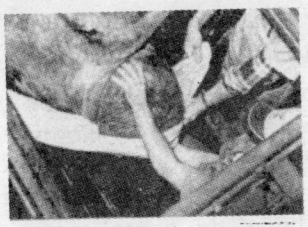

Fig. 38.6 : Replacement of a third-degree vaginal prolapse being assisted by elevation with a towel

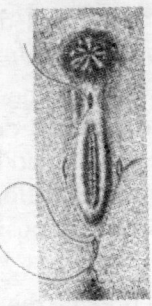

Fig. 38.7 : Method of Buhner's suture

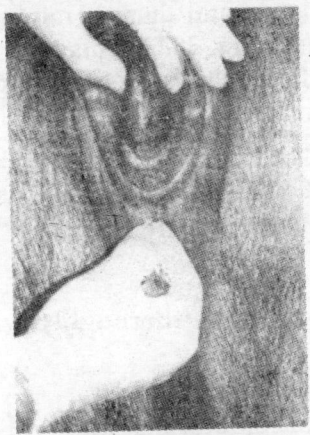

Fig. 38.8 : Stab incision in the perineum below the vulva to start the Buhner is suture

---

INTERESTING FACTS

- Once prolapse of vagina or cervix has occurred, the exposed mucus membranes as well as the vulva become very oedematous; sometimes, the urinary bladder may prolapse and continue to fill with urine. These factors prevent the return of the prolapsed structure when the cow rises (as in first-degree prolapse) and favour straining that lead to prolapse of rectum.

- Oedema of the prolapsed vagina and cervix occur because of the irritation and trauma to the exposed mucus membranes, and prolapse portion drops over the ischial arch thereby causing a passive venous congestion. This oedema tends to accumulate in the submucosa and causes separation of the mucosa from the underlying thin muscular vaginal wall.

- The prolapse of vagina in the bitches is seen most commonly at the time of oestrum unlike bovines.

Differences between third-degree vaginal prolapse or cervical prolapse in *Bos taurus* and *Bos indicus.*

- In *Bos taurus* breeds, the sequence of events leading to cervical prolapse is the same as described above. The vaginal floor and urinary bladder followed by cervix protrude through the vulva. Typically, the vaginal floor is extremely oedematous, and the external cervical os is positioned near the dorsal commissure of the vulva.

- In *Bos indicus* breeds, the cervix is prolapsed as a pedunculated mass with the external cervical os being the most distal portion of the prolapsed tissue, and there is minimal or no oedema in the vaginal floor (see Fig. 38.5). This type of prolapse usually does not progress through first or second degree, but is a primary prolapse of the cervix.

NOTE : A cow will usually calve without assistance in nearly all uncomplicated cases of first-degree prolapse and after parturition, the prolapse is usually immediately relieved.

Treatment :

1. Clean the prolapsed mass thoroughly with mild antiseptic solution.
2. Tranquillizer-siquil-5ml - I/M.
3. Administer posterior epidural anaesthesia (5-8 ml 2% lignocaine).
4. Replace the prolapsed portion.
5. Apply the xylocaine ointment inside the vaginal wall for 5 to 7 days.
6. Apply rope truss.
7. Progesterone therapy : 50 to 100 mg progesterone (Duraprogen) I/M daily or 500 mg progesterone I/M at 10 days interval. This therapy should be discontinued before the completion of gestation period.
8. Broad-spectrum antibiotics for 3-5 days.
9. Antihistaminic and multi-vitamin injections should be given parenterally.
10. Calcium injection-like COBACAL-D (Vetcare) 10ml I/M alternate day for 3-5 times.
11. Herbal preparation – **Prolapse in** 5 tab bid for 3 days.
12. Homoeopathic drug : **Opium 200** - 4-5 drops tid for 10 days.

CLINICAL POINTER

If any difficulty is encountered during the replacement of the prolapsed vagina with distended urinary bladder, the prolapsed portion should be raised dorsally to reduce the obstruction in urethra (sharp kink), thus urine comes out and urinary bladder reduces in size and now the prolapsed mass can easily be replaced or if by this method, the bladder is not reduced in size, aspirate the urine with the help of a fine needle.

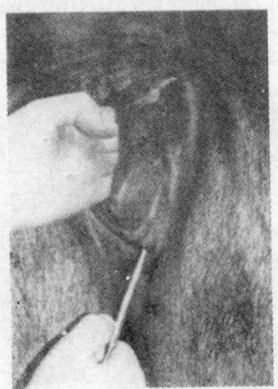

Fig. 38.9 : Passage of the Buhner needle along the constrictor vestibuli.

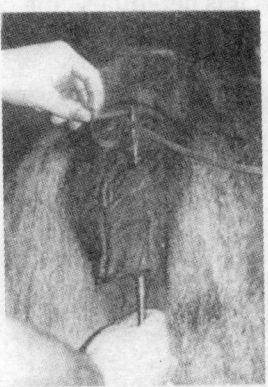

Fig. 38.10 : The Buhner needle exists the dorsal incision and Buhner tape is threaded through the eye.

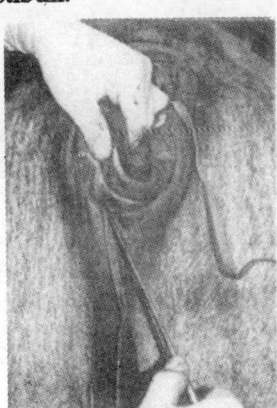

Fig. 38.11 : After the Buhner needle and tape are pulled down from first side and the needle is removed, reinsert the needle in the ventral incision and repeat the needle passage on the other side of the vulva.

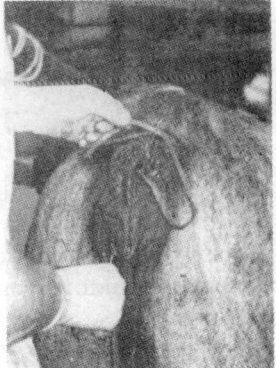

Fig. 38.12 : Thread the tail of tape on the needle. Pull the needle and tape down the final side of the vulva.

263

Advice to owner :

1) Lift the hind limbs by means of inclined platform (dig out the soil under the front quarter so that hind limb is raised by 2 to 6 inches).

2) Stop the suspected fodder (moulded feed or clover fodder).

3) Reduce the amount of feed offered to the cow.

4) Offer the **laxative feed** so that faeces will come out without straining.

5) If it is hereditary, the cow should not be used for further breeding purpose.

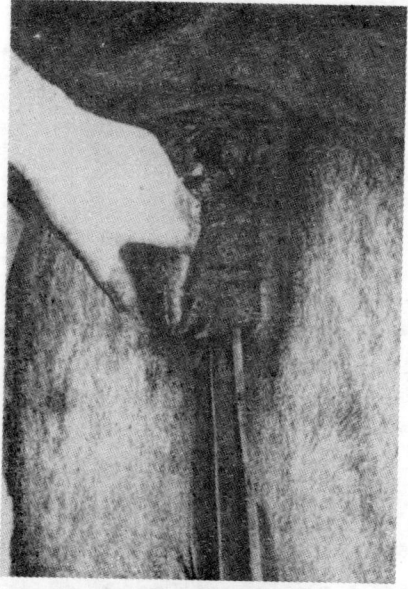 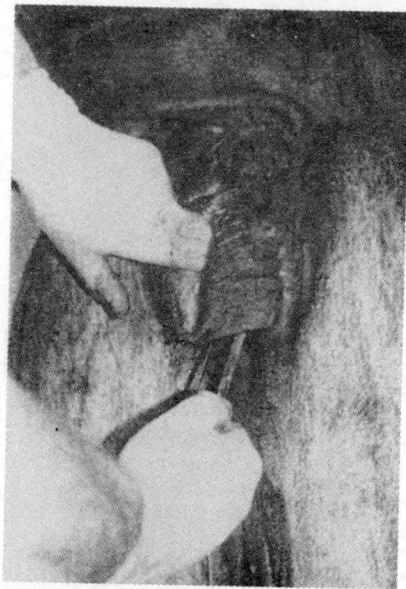

Fig. 38.13 : Suture palcement is complete, and the vulva is encompassed with two ends of the Buhner tape protruding from the ventral incision.

Fig. 38.14 : Tighten the suture such that the vestibular lumen will accommodate only two-three fingers

How to apply a rope-truss ?
• A long rope is taken.
• The middle portion of the rope is kept on the lumbo-sacral region just anterior to the tuber coxae.
• The two ends of rope are passed between the two thighs.
• A knot is made just below the ventral commissure of the vulva and is passed above the dorsal commissure by separating the two ends over the vulvar lips.
• Again a knot is made above the dorsal commissure but below the anus.
• Now the two ends of rope are passed dorsally and the ends are entangled with the loop around the lumbo-sacral region.
• One end is looped around the neck and other end is entangled to the loop.

Surgical techniques – are used after replacing the prolapsed portion in difficult chronic cases and especially when parturition is a long way ahead.

1. **Buhner's method :**
• Administer the caudal epidural anaesthesia.
• Make two horizontal incisions in the perineum just below the ventral commisure and above the dorsal commissure of vulva but below the anus (half way between the vulva and anus). see Fig. 38.7.
• Grasp the vulva with one hand and introduce the Buhner needle through the ventral incision deeply along one side of the vulva which comes out through the dorsal incision (see Fig. 38.8 and 38.9).
• Thread the Buhner tape through the eye of the needle (see Fig. 38.10).
• Forcefully pull the needle and tape ventrally, exitting through the ventral incision and remove the needle from the suture (see Fig. 38.11).
• Repeat the procedure on the opposite side of the vulva (see Fig. 38.12).

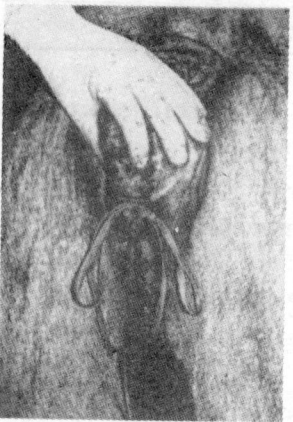 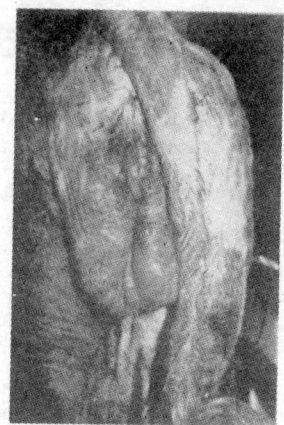

Fig. 38.15 : The the suture ends in a quick release knot to allow for rapid release during calving and for retrying afterward.

Fig. 38.16 : Vulvar oedema from a Buhner suture. It is a complication with Buhner procedure. In the indigenous cows with an extremely pendulous vulva, placement of suture may create severe oedema of the vulva.

- Apply traction to the two ends of the suture tape to reduce the vulvar lumen so that it can accommodate only one or two fingers (see Fig. 38.13 and 38.14).

- Tie the ends of the suture tape in either a square knot or quick-release knot (see Fig. 38.15).

NOTE : The advantage of the quick-release knot is that the suture may be untied during calving and then re-tied without total replacement, if there is any chance of post-partum prolapse.

INTERESTING FACT
Advantages of Buhner's method are that this is the most physiological method of retention of prolapsed mass because the suture mimics the constrictor vestibuli muscle and there is minimal deformation of vulva.

2. **Caslick operation (Vulvoplasty) :**

- Administer epidural anaesthesia or local infiltration (see Fig. 38.17).

- Remove the mucus membrane 1.2 cm wide with the help of scissors from the upper 3/4th of each vulvar lip (see Fig. 38.18).

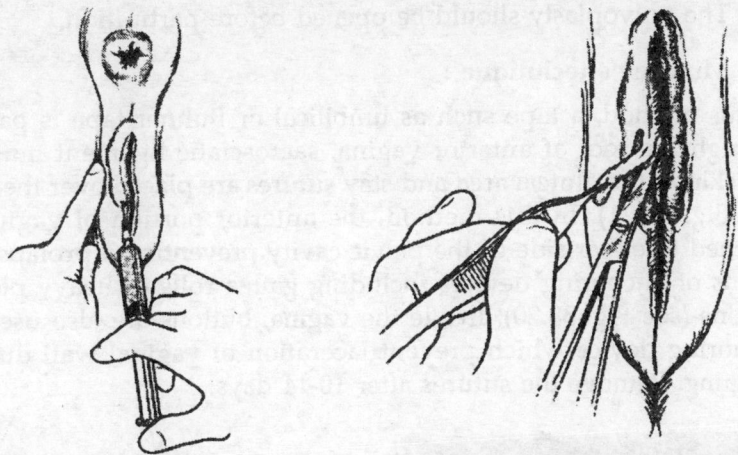

Fig. 38.17 : Local infiltration of anaesthetic agents for Caslick's procedure. **Fig. 38.18 : Removal of narrow strip of tissue from muco-cutaneous junction with scissors.**

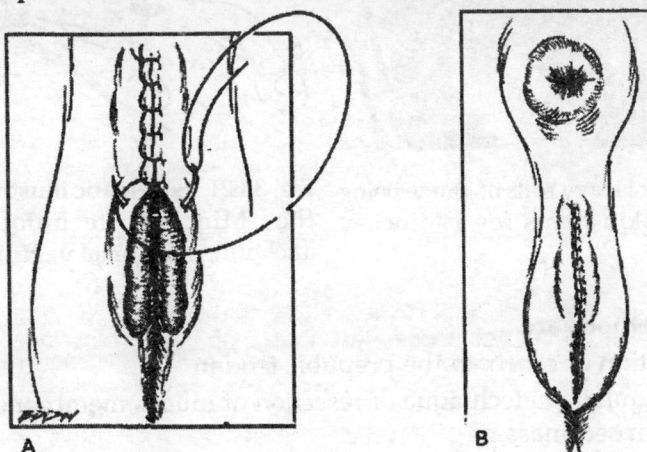

A   B

Fig. 38.19 : A and B. Closure of Caslick's vulvoplasty using continuous interlocking system

- Close the denuded area using continuous interlocking pattern by means of fine nylon sutures (see Fig. 38.19).
- One or two deep horizontal mattress vulvar sutures of umbilical tape are placed through the skin 2 to 3 inches lateral to the vulva to protect the lip from tearing during straining.
- After 10 days, all sutures should be removed.
- Now the vulvar opening is so small that the vaginal wall cannot prolapse.

- The vulvoplasty should be opened before parturition.

3. Minchev's technique :

In this method, a tape such as umbilical or Buhner tape is passed through the roof of anterior vagina, sacrosciatic ligament muscles and skin in the gluteal area and stay sutures are placed over the skin (see Fig. 38.21). In this method, the anterior portion of vagina is fastened to either side of the pelvic cavity preventing a prolapse by means of anchoring devices including gauze rolls or heavy plastic buttons (see Fig. 38.20). Inside the vagina, buttons are also used as anchoring device which prevent laceration of vaginal wall during straining. Remove the sutures after 10-14 days.

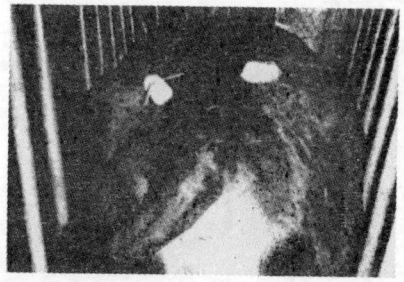

Fig. 38.20 : Heavy rolls of gauze being used as skin stents for a Minchev technique.

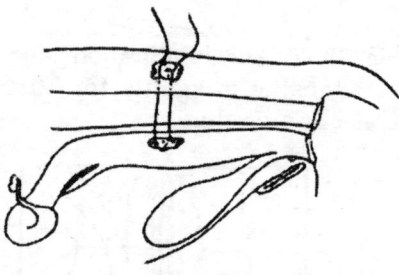

Fig. 38.21 : Schematic illustration of the Minchev technique for anchoring the dorsal vagina

Other methods are :

- Fixation of cervix to the prepubic tendon .
- Faraquharson technique of resection of mucus membrane of the prolapsed mass.
- Removal of perivaginal fat.
- Pumping of air into peritoneum.

CLINICAL POINTER

If constant tenesmus or straining after replacement of the prolapsed mass is present, then repeated dose of caudal epidural anaesthesia at one to two hours 'interval may be helpful after fixing the needle in sacro-coccygeal region with the help of tape. In this condition, use of lignocaine and xylazine combination may be more useful. For details see the chapter "caudal epidural anaesthesia."

OBSERVATIONS :

Date ....

- Case No. ....
- Species ....
- Age ....
- History ....
- Offered feed and fodder ....
- Conformation of animal ....
- About exercise of animal ....
- Stage of gestation ....
- Temperature ....
- Pulse rate ....
- Feed and water intake ....
- Local anaesthetic used ....
- Dose of local anaesthetic ....
- Method employed to replace the prolapsed mass ....
- Method employed to retain the prolapsed part ....

1. Treatment given

   Rx

   1. ....
   2. ....
   3. ....
   4. ....

Prognosis ....

EXERCISE :

1. What is the main reason for vaginal prolapse ?

Ans.

2. What are the main features of third-degree prolapse ?

Ans.

3. What are the reasons which prevent the prolapsed mass to return when a cow rises from sitting position ?

Ans.

4. In which stage, prolapse of vagina in the bitch is most commonly found ?

Ans.

5. What will be your tentative diagnosis when a cow has scars on the vulva?

Ans.

6. What are the advantages of Buhner's method ?

ns.

7. What are the advantages of fixation of cervix to the prepubic tendon ?

Ans.

8. What is principle of pumping air into peritoneum during the treatment of prolapse of vagina ?

Ans.

�֎ ✖ ✖ ✖ ✖

The wind and the waves are always on the side of the ablest navigators.
– Edward Gibbon

Chapter 39

Diagnosis and Therapeutic Management of Uterine Prolapse in Bovines

Prolapse or eversion of the uterus :
- It is also called **casting of "wethers"** or **casting of the "calf-bed"**.
- It occurs immediately after parturition or occasionally upto several hours or days afterwards.

Causes :
- Hypocalcaemia
- Violent or strong tenesmus
- Relaxed, atonic and flaccid uterus
- Retention of placenta especially at the ovarian end of gravid horn
- Excessive relaxation of the pelvic and perineal regions
- Inadequate exercise
- Vigorous force applied during forced traction of foetus

Clinical signs :
- If recently prolapsed, it is warm to touch but later becomes cold and discoloured.
- The uterus may be grossly contaminated and lacerated.
- Mucus membrane of uterus with its cotyledons remains exposed.
- Enlarged and oedematous.
- In most animals, prolapse of uterus results in mild to moderate symptoms of tenesmus, restlessness, pain, anxiety, anorexia, increased pulse rate and respiration rate.
- The cow may be standing or recumbent.
- Death may occur due to internal haemorrhage as a result of the excessive tension placed on arteries by the prolapsed mass.

271

Treatment : (A) Replacement of uterus :

- Caudal epidural anaesthesia is administered (5-8 ml).

- The uterus should be supported by towel or a piece of board about 1 meter long covered by a clean cloth or towel at the level of vulva or ischial arch.

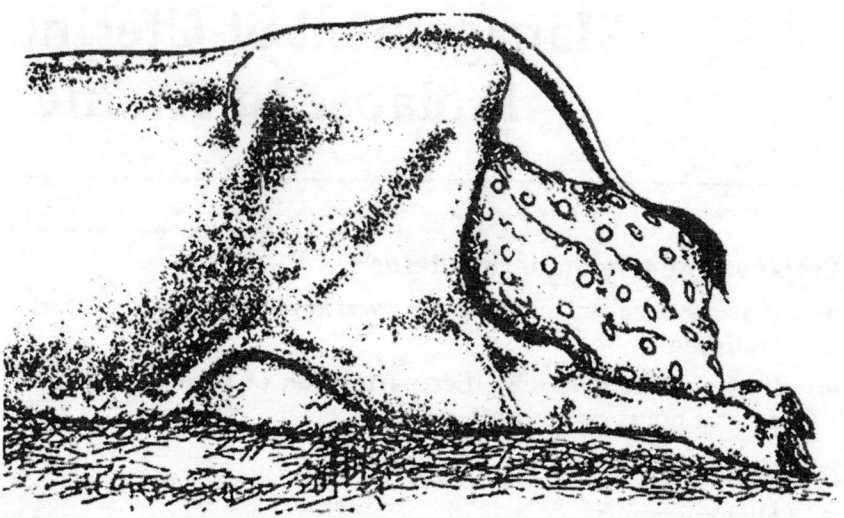

Fig. 39.1 : Cow-uterine prolapse, patient positioned for replacement. (Courtesy of Jackson, P.G.G. 1995. Handbook of Veterinary Obstetrics. W.B. Saunders Company Limited).

- Clean the uterus with water containing mild antiseptic (potassium permaganate etc.).

- Remove the placenta from the cotyledons – if it separates easily. If not, leave it attached.

- Repair any gross damage such as tearing by using an absorbable suture.

- Replace the uterus little by little with those portions nearest to the vulvar lips.

- First the ventral portion and then the dorsal portion of the prolapsed mass should be replaced.

Precaution : During the replacement of the uterus, pressure should be exerted with the help of palm and extended fingers, to prevent injury to the uterus because if accidentally cotyledons get reptured, profuse bleeding may occur.

- As the prolapsed mass comes inside the lips of the vulva, use fist to press the prolapsed mass through the cervix to the full length of arm until the gravid horn becomes straight and no invagination remains present.
- If invagination is still present, hold the **"wine bottle" with its neck and insert the hand and press the invaginated portion.**
- During pressing the clenched fist, cervix should be pulled toward him or herself with one hand.
- As soon as the uterus is replaced, the hand should be kept in the uterus and the assistant should be told to inject 20-30 IU oxytocin i/m. This will help the uterus and cervix to get contracted. When the cervix starts contracting, the hand should be removed.
- According to many researchers, temporary suturing of the vulva or application of a rope-truss is merely a placebo for the farmer because very rarely, a prolapse of uterus recur if the uterus is properly replaced.

(B) Post-replacement care :
- Antibiotic coverage especially oxytetracycline for 5 to 7 days
- Non-Steroidal anti-inflammatory drugs (NSAIDS)
- Anti-histaminics
- Vitamin B-complex inj. for 5 days
- Tranquillizer siquil-5 ml. I/M
- Application of lignocaine ointment on the vaginal wall 2 to 3 times for 3-4 days.
- Good nursing
- Light diet
- Moderate exercise
- Hind limbs should be raised.

CLINICAL POINTER

If the cow continues straining following replacement of the uterus, it may be due to invagination of the ovarian end of uterine horn or an irritation or inflammation of the vulva. The invagination can be corrected by inserting the clenched fist again. The irritation can be abolished by applying the lignocaine ointment on the vulva.

New Zealand method
When the prolapsed mass is so large that it is impossible to replace it back its original position in standing condition of cow, then the cow is placed in sternal recumbency with her hind legs pulled out behind her (see Fig. 39.1). Two or three assistants are required for this. She must be cast on her side and the uppermost hind limb pulled out behind her. She is then rolled on to her other side so that the second hind limb may be secured and extended caudally. The obstetrician should kneel down behind the cow and takes the prolapsed mass on his or her lap and then the uterus is replaced slowly. Replacement is greatly helped if the cow's hind quarters are higher than her fore quarters.

OBSERVATIONS :

Date ....

- Case No. ....
- Species ....
- Age ....
- History ....
- Symptoms ....
- Size of prolapsed mass ....
- Conditions of prolapsed mass *contaminated/lacerated/warm to touch/ cold/ discoloured.*
- Condition of placenta – *easily separated / not easily separated.*
- Repair of any gross damage – *Yes/No.*
- Replacement procedure ....
  ....
  ....
  ....

- Post-operative treatment and care

Rx.

1.

2.

3.

4.

Prognosis ....

EXERCISE :

1. What do you mean by the casting of 'Wether' ?
Ans.

2. What is the common cause of death in prolapse of uterus ?
Ans.

3. How will you diagnose the case of recently prolapsed uterus ?
Ans.

4. The prolapsed mass is kept at the level of ischial arch or vulva during replacement. Give reason.
Ans.

5. Enlist the methods to keep the prolapsed mass at the level of ischial arch ?
Ans.

6. Which portion of the prolapsed mass should be replaced first ?
Ans.

7. The wine bottle is used to replace the uterus. Give reason.
Ans.

8. What may be the reasons of straining of a cow after replacement of uterus ?
Ans.

9. After replacement of uterus, how much time is taken to close the cervix ?
Ans.

10. What is the New Zealand method ?
Ans.

❈ ❈ ❈ ❈ ❈

Opportunities are usually disguised as hard work, so most people do not recognize them.

Chapter 40

Diagnosis and Therapeutic Management of Foetal Mummification

Definition : *"The process in which a foetus dies within the uterus, autolysis occurs without putrefaction and the remaining shrivelled mass of bones gets usually enclosed in wrinkled brown skin is known as foetal mummification."*

INTERESTING FACT
Foetal mummification does not occur in the first trimester of pregnancy because embryonic or foetal death occurring before the development of foetal bones is usually absorbed.

Susceptible animals : Foetal mummification is commonly found in cattle and pigs than sheep, horses, dogs and cats.

Causes of foetal mummification :

Bovines :

- **Genetic and chromosomal abnormalities** (common in Jersey breed of cattle).

- It may be due to **torsion of umbilical cord or compression of the umbilical cord.** Hence, blood supply is obstructed and the foetus dies.

- There is evidence that foetal mummification may follow infectious causes of foetal death such as *Campylobacter foetus*, moulds, *leptospira* spp. and Bovine Viral Diarrhoea (BVD) virus.

Swine :

- Many viruses can cross the maternal placenta and kill the conceptus. Dead embryos are usually absorbed without a trace, whereas foetuses i.e. the conceptus after about 30 days of gestational age when skeletal development begins, will either dehydrated (mummified) or aborted. These viruses are porcine parvovirus (PPV), porcine enterovirus (PEV), Japanese B encephalitis virus etc.

- Uterine over-crowding and placental insufficiency.
- In multiparous animals, due to more litters, over-crowding of uterus occurs which results in deficiencies of placenta to some foetuses and the foetus dies.

Ewe: Foetal mummification is generally found with twins or triplets when one of the embryos has died.

Mare: Mummification is rare and is always associated with twin pregnancies. If twinning occurs, one of the foetuses usually develops more slowly than the other. The smaller foetus usually dies. The dead foetus will be mummified and delivered at term with live foal.

Bitch: In the bitch, foetal mummification is a characteristic of *canine herpes virus infection.*

Queen: It is not uncommon in cat and is assumed to be due to uterine overcrowding.

Types of foetal mummification :

There are two types of foetal mummification.

(i) Haematic mummification :

This type of mummification is found in **cattle**. After the foetal death, involution of caruncles occur which result in variable amount of haemorrhages between the endometrium and foetal membranes. The plasma of the blood is absorbed, only RBCs remain present. Haemoglobin, as a result of haemolysis of the RBCs, stain reddish-brown colour to the foetal membrane and the foetus. Therefore, this type of mummification is called haematic mummification.

Foetal mummification occurs when a foetus dies without luteolysis and adequate cervical dilatation. *A functional corpus luteum is a cardinal feature of the condition.* Mummification occurs as a result of autolysis of foetal tissue and fluid absorption in a sterile environment.

(ii) Papyraceous mummification : This type of mummification is generally found in the *sow, bitch* and *cat.* In this type of mummification, placental haemorrhage does not occur, so there is no reddish-brown staining of the foetal membranes. The mummified foetus is usually brownish in colour. Here, foetal fluid is absorbed and foetal membranes become shrivelled and dried, so that it **resemble a parchment**. Hence this type of mummification is called papyraceous mummification.

DO YOU KNOW ?
Previously, it was thought that foetal death occurs due to caruncular haemorrhage but now it is thought that haemorrhage is effect of foetal death rather than its cause.

Differences between Haematic and papyraceous mummification :

Haematic mummification	Papyraceous mummification
1. Only found in cattle	1. Commonest form.
2. Foetal membranes remain surrounded by a viscous, chocolate-coloured material.	2. Foetal membranes remain contracted, wrinkled and dried like parchment.
3. Foetal membrane is reddish-brown in colour due to pigments from RBCs.	3. Foetal membrane is brownish in colour.
4. Caruncular haemorrhage occurs.	4. No caruncular haemorrhage occurs.

MUMMIFICATION AND CORPUS LUTEUM
• In bovines and rarely in goat, foetal mummification is associated with persistent corpus luteum. The mummified foetus does not give any signal for onset of parturition (normally mature foetus, at the end of gestation, give signal through *hypothalamus-pituitary-adrenal axis* for onset of parturition). So corpus luteum remains present and also mummified foetus remains present in the uterus for indefinite time (prolonged gestation). • In other species, progesterone is produced by the placenta after mid-gestation, so normally corpora lutea regress. In this way, during mummification in other species, persistent corpus luteum is not a characteristic as in the case of cattle.

Clinical signs and diagnosis (in bovines) :

1.   Mummification may be suspected when a cow is believed to be pregnant but fails to show abdominal or mammary enlargement near her expected term.

2.   **Rectal palpation :**

● The gravid horn appears tightly surrounding the foetus.

● *In some large cows, the foetus may be out of reach from examiner's hand because uterus remains intra-abdominal.* For this two assistants are required, they raise the caudal abdomen of the cow with the help of a plank which brings the foetus within reach during rectal palpation.

● Fluidity in the horn is not palpable as in normal pregnancy.

● No fremitus is detectable in the middle uterine artery.

● The cotyledons are not palpable.

● **Persistent corpus luteum.**

● Uterine wall becomes fairly thick.

MUMMIFICATION AND GESTATION PERIOD
The bovine mummified foetus usually remains in the uterus without odour or pus until the condition is diagnosed and treated while in other domestic animals mummified foetus usually remain in the uterus only as long as pregnancy is maintained by other viable foetuses and expelled with normal foetuses at the time of parturition.

Treatment :

1.   **Administration of PGF$_2\alpha$ analogue :** The treatment of choice is a single injection of PGF$_2\alpha$ analogue. The PGF$_2\alpha$ analogue causes regression of CL. After regression of CL, new follicles develop and the cow comes in heat, the cervix opens and the mummified foetus passes out from the uterus and lodges usually in the vagina within 4 days. A second treatment is rarely necessary.

   Lutalyse (Dinoprost) – 5 ml (25 mg) I/M or Vetmate (cloprostenol) – 2ml – I/M

2.   **Administration of oestradiol valerate :** Intramuscular injection of oestradiol causes contraction of the uterine muscles, relaxation of the cervix, regression of the corpus luteum and expulsion of the foetus. If the foetus is not expelled after 72 hours (3 days), same dose should be administered again.

   Progynon-depot (oestradiol valerate)- 1 ml I/M

279

> ### CLINICAL POINTER
>
> Whether prostaglandins or oestrogens are used, expulsion of the mummified foetus may not be complete because of poor dilatation and dryness of the cervix and birth-canal. Lubrication of the birth-canal and traction are required for the delivery of the mummified foetus in some cases.

3. If the mummified foetus is very large or previous treatment has failed, then caesarean operation should be done.

4. Since there is sterile environment of uterus, there is no need of antibiotic therapy either systemically or locally. But when during manual traction, injury of birth-canal occurs and/or there are chances of entry of infection, then antibiotic should be administered.

5. After expulsion of mummified foetus, vitamin A and phosphorus inj. should be administered to restore the uterine epithelial cells and for increasing the tone of the uterus.

Prognosis :

*   After expulsion of foetus, most cows recover quickly since no infection is present. Thus prognosis for rebreeding of the female is good. Most cases will conceive 1 to 3 months after expulsion of a mummified foetus.

*   Any cow with a history of having one mummified calf may have another one at any gestation period (if mummification is due to genetical)

Advice : If the condition is hereditary in nature, cull the bull or the cow after identification.

OBSERVATIONS :

Date : ....

*   Case No. ....
*   Species ....
*   Breed ....
*   Age ....
*   Date of last service ....
*   *Per-rectal* examination ....
    Fremitus   *Present/Absent*
    Cotyledons   *Present/Absent*

Uterine wall	*Thick/Thin*
Fluidity in the horn	*Present/Absent*
Horns	*Within reach/Out of reach*
Cervix	*Stretched/Normal*
Corpus luteum	*Present/Absent*

- Diagnosis ....
- **Treatment**

  Rx

  1.

  2.

  3.

  4.

EXERCISE :

1. Mummification does not occur in the first trimester of pregnancy. Give reason.

Ans.

2. In which species mummification is commonly found ?

Ans.

3. Enlist the causes of mummification of foetuses in bovine.

Ans.

4. Enlist the causes of mummification of foetuses in swine.

Ans.

5. What is the most common cause of mummification of foetus in equine ?

Ans.

6. What is the most common cause of mummification of foetus in canine ?

Ans.

7. Which type of mummification is found in bovine ?

Ans.

8. Which type of mummification is found in swine ?

Ans.

9. What is the reason of reddish-brown stain of the foetal membranes of mummified foetus of bovine ?

Ans.

10. Mummification in swine is called papyraceous mummification. Give reason.

Ans.

11. Mummification in bovine is called haematic mummification. Give reason.

Ans.

12. Why does corpus luteum remain present in case of bovine mummification?

Ans.

13. Why are persistant corpora lutea not present in case of swine mummification?

Ans.

14. How does $PGF_2\alpha$ analogue help in expulsion of mummified foetus ?

Ans.

15. Why mummified foetus should be removed with care from vagina by gentle traction using plenty of lubrication ?

Ans.

�֍ ✶ ✶ ✶ ✶

Replace positive thinking with positive doing.

Chapter 41

Diagnosis and Therapeutic Management of Foetal Maceration

Definition : *"The process in which a foetus dies after ossification within the uterus and the foetus undergoes microbial digestion or putrefaction in the fluid of uterus till only the mass of bones remains, is known as maceration."*

Foetal maceration can occur in any species, but it is described most frequently in cattle.

Pathogenesis
• Foetal maceration can take place at any stage of gestation but can only be detected when death occurs after 3 months of age (bovines) because, if foetal death occurs before ossification of the bones, complete microbial digestion of foetus occurs followed by pyometra. • When death of foetus occur due to bacterial or viral infections, there may or may not be regression of corpus luteum. The parturient phenomenon is initiated but the abortion is incomplete due to incomplete dilatation of the cervical canal. The foetus undergoes microbial digestion in the fluid of uterus till only the mass of bones remains. The causative organisms are normally those found in the uterus. The micro-organisms get a favorable environment due to patent cervix and optimum temperature and multiply rapidly. Sometimes, the foetal bones penetrate the uterine wall and cause severe damage to the endometrium.

Clinical signs :
• Intermittent straining for several days accompanied by a foul, foetid, reddish-grey vulvar discharge.
• Pulse and temperature elevated

- Anorexia
- Drop in milk production
- Diarhoea occasionally

On per rectal examination :

- **Metallic sound or gritty feeling** due to sliding movement of bones on each other after complete maceration of foetus.
- No fremitus in the middle uterine artery is detectable

In long-standing cases :

- No straining
- Cervix is usually quite contracted
- No elevated pulse and temperature
- No anorexia
- Foetid and muco-purulent discharge from vulva
- Metallic sound or gritty feeling on per rectal examination

Treatment :

1. Manual removal of foetus or foetal part (s) when cervix is dilated.
2. When cervix is partially open, then cervix dilatating drug can be administered. Epidosin vet (Velethamide bromide) – 5 ml (50 mg) – I/M
3. PGF$_2\alpha$ or oestrogen is also given for cervical relaxation.
4. After cervical relaxation, all the foetal parts and bones are removed carefully so that no foetal bone remains present in the uterus.
5. **Oxytocin should not be given in case of maceration because it increases the contractibility of the uterus** and if some bones are left even after manual removal, these penetrate the uterus and cause peritonitis etc.
6. Large doses of antibiotics should be given parenterally as well as intrauterine preferably oxytetracycline for 4 to 5 days.

   For intrauterine therapy, 4-8 boluses of terramycin are dissolved in 30-40 ml sterile water.

   Lixen (cephalexin) intrauterine is also beneficial, 4.5 gm powder is dissolved in 60 ml sterile water and infusee in the uterus for 4-5 days.

7. **Supportive therapy :**

   (a) **Vit. A injection :** For restoration of endometrial epithelial cells.

   (b) **Tonophosphan :** 10 ml I/M alternate day for 3 days.

   (c) **Vitamin B-complex with liver extract :** 10 ml I/M for 3-5 days.

   (d) **Fluid therapy :** In severe condition toxaemia cause septic shock and lactic acidosis. Therefore, a cow needs balanced isotonic, alkalinizing multiple electrolyte infusion in large volumes.

   Rintose – 1 litre I/V daily for 3 to 4 days.

Differences between mummification and maceration :

Mummification	Maceration
1. Corpus luteum present	1. Corpus luteum generally absent.
2. Uterus is not invaded by putrefying bacteria	2. Uterus is invaded by putrefying bacteria.
3. Cervix remains closed	3. Generally cervix remains dilated
4. No vaginal discharge	4. Foul, foetid and reddish-grey vaginal discharge.
5. No straining	5. Straining
6. No elevation of temperature and pulse.	6. Elevation of temperature and pulse.
7. Normal appetite	7. Anorexia
8. No drop in milk production.	8. Drop in milk production
9. On per-rectal examination gravid horn appears tightly surrounding the foetus.	9. Metallic sound or gritty feeling due to sliding of bones on each other when examined per-rectally

Prognosis : Future breeding life of cattle is very questionable. The longer the condition has existed, the greater the damage to the endometrium and poorer the prognosis.

OBSERVATIONS :

Date.....................

- Case No. ....
- Species ....
- Breed ....
- Age of animal ....
- Number of calving ....
- Date of last service...............................
- General conditions

Temperature ....
Pulse rate ....
Appetite ....
Ruminal motility ....
Vaginal discharge..........................
Digestive problem ....
Any other symptoms ....
• Per-rectal examination finding (s)

‒ ‒
‒ ‒
‒ ‒

• Diagnosis ....
• **Treatment**
   Rx
       1.
       2.
       3.
       4.

EXERCISE :

1. What happens when foetal death occurs before 3 months of gestation in bovine ?

Ans.

2. Diarrhoea occurs sometimes in case of maceration of foetus. Give reason.

Ans.

3. Why 'metallic sound' or 'grity feeling' is found during per-rectal examination of maceration of foetus ?

Ans.

4. Why oxytocin is not generally given in case of maceration?

Ans.

❈ ❈ ❈ ❈ ❈

Do not be afraid of defeat. You are never so near to victory as when defeated in a good cause.
– H.W. Beecher

Chapter 42

Diagnosis and Therapeutic Management of Hydramnios and Hydrallantois

Hydramnios or hydrops of the amnion :

It is characterized by gradual enlargement of the amniotic cavity due to excessive accumulation of amniotic fluid in the last half of the gestation. It 's common in cattle and buffalo.

Physiopathology
The source of the amniotic fluid in early and mid-gestation is secretion of amniotic epithelium and foetal urine. As gestation advances, the allantoic fluid increases in volume while the amniotic fluid remains fairly static but becomes viscid and mucoid because urinary bladder sphincter prevents further release of the urine into the amniotic cavity. Now, the source of the mucoid amniotic fluid after mid-gestation is saliva and secretion of the naso-pharynx of the foetus because a large volume of saliva is continually produced after mid-gestation. Swallowing of fluid by the foetus controls the volume of amniotic fluid. In this way, volume of amniotic fluid remains static after mid-gestation (2 to 8 litres with an average of 5 litres).
When genetically or congenital-defective foetus (like cleft palate, schistosoma reflexus etc) remains in uterus, swallowing is affected and the volume of amniotic fluid gradually starts to accumulate upto **8-10 times i.e. 20 to 100 litres.** This condition is called hydramnios.

Cause : Genetical or congenital-defective foetus which is unable to swallow the fluid.

Symptoms :
- Slow enlargement of abdomen.

- **Pear-shaped abdomen.**
- Often, the condition is not recognized during pregnancy but at the time of parturition, large quantities of syrupy and viscid amniotic fluid is released. The fluid often contains **meconium.**
- Foetus is either dead or if **delivered alive,** does not survive.
- Pregnancy may continue but **dystocia** occurs due to ineffective labour.

INTERESTING FACT
Since the abdominal wall has more time to adjust the gradually increasing weight and volume, so the abdomen becomes pear-shaped and less tense than that of a cow with hydrallantois in which suddenly or within short period of time, fluid gets accumulated.

Hydrallantois or Hydrops of the allantois :

It is characterized by Sudden enlargement of the allantoic sac due to excessive accumulation of allantoic fluid within a period of 5 to 20 days in late gestation. It is common in cattle and buffalo.

Physiopathology
Initially, the small amount of allantoic fluid remains present in the allantoic sac from the allantoic epithelium or by absorption from the uterine lumen. The large volume of allantoic fluid starts to accumulate after the formation of kidney. Thus, allantoic cavity stores the waste products of the foetal kidney. This fluid is **clear, watery and amber in colour.** As the pregnancy advances, the volume of allantoic fluid also increases. Towards the end of gestation, volume of the fluid varies from **4 to 15 litres, average 9.5 litres in normal cow.** The outer layer of the allantois is richly supplied with blood vessels connected to the foetus by the umbilical arteries and umbilical vein.   Occasionally, excessive amount of allantoic fluid (**80 to 150 litres or more**) accumulate in the allantoic cavity. **The excessive fluid is similar in nature to transudate indicating vascular disturbance in the allantois.**

Causes :

- It is usually associated with a **diseased uterus** in which most of the caruncles in one horn are not functional and the rest of the placentomes are greatly enlarged and possibly, the diseased uterus causes **vascular disturbances.**

- Adventitious placentae and twin foetuses are commonly associated with hydrallantois.

DO YOU KNOW ?	
Dropsy of Foetal Sacs	**Dropsy of Foetus**
• Hydramnios	• Hydrocephalus
• Hydrallantois	• Foetal ascites
	• Foetal anasarca

Symptoms :
- **Barrel-shaped abdomen**
- Anorexia
- Dehydration
- Weakness
- Difficulty in respiration due to abdominal distension
- Placentomes and foetus are not palpable on per rectal examination
- Sudden increase in weight and volume of the uterus predisposes the females to **ventral hernia**
- Temperature normal but pulse elevated
- **Drink excessive amount of water**
- The cow loses body condition and lastly becomes unable to rise
- Dislocation of hips may occur and the cow lies on her sternum looking like a **bloated bull-frog**

Differences between hydrallantois and hydramnios

Points	Hydrallantois	Hydramnios
1. Incidence	85 to 90%	5 to 10%
2. Abdominal enlargement	Rapid within 5 to 20 days	Slowly over months.
3. Abdominal shape	Barrel-shaped and tense	Pear-shaped and less tense
4. Volume of fluid	80-150 litres or more (Normal 9.5 litres)	20-100 litres (Normal 5 litres)
5. Fluid characteristics	Watery, clean and amber coloured with characteristics of transduate	Viscid and syrupy and often contain meconium.
6. Foetus	Small and not palpable	Defective foetus and palpable

7. Horns	Palpable	Difficult to palpate
8. Placentomes	Not palpable, less in number & hypertrophic.	Palpable & normal
9. Chorioallantois	Diseased	Normal
10. Abdominal hernia	Common in severe cases	Rare
11. Uterine rupture	Common	Uncommon
12. Retained placenta	Common	Occasional
13. Prognosis	**Guarded to poor** for life and fertility	**Fair to good** for life and fertility

CLINICAL POINTER

An owner believes that either his/her records of breeding date is wrong or the cow has twins or triplets by seeing the excessive distension of abdomen. Later, he/she gets confused with digestive problems because anorexia, lack of rumination and constipation are noted. This condition is frequently misdiagnosed with indigestion, bloat or traumatic gastritis. Therefore, a clinician should always do per rectal examination carefully.

INTERESTING FACT

The lack of caruncles predispose the cow to hydrallantois. Therefore, it occurs in the cows which are old because in old cows, less caruncles remain present due to prior uterine infection or tuberculous metritis. This condition is seen in heifers due to congenital lack of caruncles rarely.

Treatment :

- If the cow is bright and active, there is no need for specific treatment but assistance may be required at the time of calving because parturition is usually abnormal.

- If the cow is in distress, it is necessary to terminate the pregnancy by one of the methods mentioned below :

  - $PGF_2\alpha$ analogues one to two times induce the parturition.

  - Parturition can also be induced with single or repeated treatment of 20 to 40 mg **dexamethasone injection**.

  - Pregnancy can be reliably terminated in 24 to 48 hours with simultaneous injection of 25 mg **dexamethosone** and $PGF_2\alpha$ **analogue** (Lutalyse, 5 ml).

  - 20 mg **dexamethasone injection** relaxes the cervix within 4 to 5 days then **oxytocin** intravenous drip for 30 minutes also give good result.

- Most severely affected cows remain dehydrated with marked electrolyte imbalance. **Large volumes of intravenous fluid** (rintose or intalyte) are required for several days to maintain hydration.

- When abdominal distension is severe enough to cause respiratory difficulty, fluid should be drained out from the uterus. A catheter should be aseptically placed with a surgical approach via the right flank.

- Parenteral antibiotics should be continued during and after the treatment until the placenta is passed and the uterus begins to involute.

OBSERVATIONS :

Date ....

- Case No. ....
- Species ....
- Age of Animal.............................
- Number of calving....................,........
- Stage of gestation ....
- Pulse rate ....
- Temperature rate ....
- Respiration ....
- Appetite   *Normal/Reduce/Complete anorexia.*
- Water intake   *Normal/Excess/Reduced*
- Rumination   *Normal/Reduce/Completely absent*
- Shape of abdomen   *Barrel-shaped/Pear-shaped*

Findings of per-rectal examination :
- Foetus   *Palpable/Not palpable*
- Placentomes   *Palpable/Not palpable*
- Size of placentomes   *Normal/Enlarged*
- Fremitus   *Present/Absent*
- Other findings if any ....
- Diagnosis ....
- Prognosis ....
- **Treatment**

Rx
1.
2.
3.
4.

EXERCISE :

1. What is the cause of hydramnios ?

Ans.

2. What is the cause of hydrallantois ?

Ans.

3. Distended abdomen is barrel-shaped in the case of hydrallantois. Why ?

Ans.

4. Distended abdomen is pear-shaped in the case of hydramnios. Why ?

Ans

6. What is the reason of difficult breathing in case of severe hydrallantois ?

Ans.

7. What is the volume of amniotic fluid in case of hydramnios ?

Ans.

8. What is the volume of allantoic fluid in case of hydrallantois ?

Ans.

9. Which is the most common form of dropsy of the foetal sacs ?

Ans.

�֎ ✖ ✖ ✖ ✖

A good speech has a good beginning and a good ending, both of which are kept very close together.

Chapter 43

Artificial Induction of Lactation in Infertile Bovine

Induction of lactation :

There are various methods to induce lactation in infertile cows by using oestrogen-progesterone combination.

First method :

Steps :

1. **1st day to 3rd days :**

    (a) Stilboestrol (Vetoestrol, M & B, Mumbai)

    Dose : 30 mg (total dose) S/C daily.

    (b) Hydroxy progesterone (Duraprogen, Vetcare)

    Dose:- 250 mg. or 1ml. (total dose) I/M daily.

2. **4th day to 7th days :**

    (a) Stilboestrol (Vetoestrol, M & B Mumbai)

    Dose: 20 mg. (total dose) S/C daily.

    (b) Hydroxy progesterone (Duraprogen, Vetcare)

    Dose:- 250 mg or 1ml (total dose) I/M daily.

3. **8th and 9th days:-**

    Stilboestrol

    Dose 20 mg S/C daily.

4. **10th to 14th days:-**

    Contraceptive pills used in human practice containing.

    Norethisterone 1mg and Ethinyl estradiol 30 mg. per tablet (MALA-N,IOPL Gurgaon) to maintain oestrogen concentration in the blood.

    Dose :- 1 tablet per day orally.

5. **11th to 15th days :-**

   Dexamethasone

   Dose 5ml I/M daily.

6. The udder and teats are massaged twice daily for 5 minutes till the flow of milk started.

   - The mammary glands develop gradually up to the 8th days and then faster upto 11th days.

   - On milking, watery fluid starts to come out which turn milky in appearance after administration of dexamethasone.

   - After the induction of lactation, initially the milk has unpleasant odour, taste, and it curdles on boiling. Probably this is due to steroid secretion in the milk. This milk should not be used for human consumption.

   - After nearly 20 days, the flavour and taste of the milk improves, the curdling disappears and now it is fit for consumption.

Second method :

Steps :

Deworming should be done before starting the treatment.

1. **1st day :-**

   (a) Stilboestrol

   Dose : 25 mg (total dose) – S/C

   (b) Hydroxy progesterone

   Dose : 250 mg (total dose) I/M.

2. **2nd day :-**

   (a) Repeat **Stilboestrol** + Hydroxy-progesterone

   (b) Lactomag (calcium borogluconate)

   Dose : 450 ml. slow I/V

   (c) Hermin (Amino acid infusions)

   Dose : 200 ml I/V

3. **4th to 10th days.**

   - Repeat Stilboestrol and Hydroxy-progesterone.

   - From 7th day, milk like discharge starts to come out.

   - On the 10th day, about 100 ml. milk can be procured.

4. 11th to 13th days :-

(a) Metaclopromide (Perinorm)

Dose : 10 mg or 2 ml (total dose) I/M daily

(b) Prednisolone

Dose : 20 mg or 2 ml (total dose) I/M daily

The udder and teats are massaged twice daily for 5 minutes after starting the treatment.

Third method :

On the '0' day :-

oestradiol valerate (Progynon depot)

Dose : 1ml – I/M

On the 7th day :-

Cloprostenol sodium (Vetmate)

Dose : 2 ml – I/M

On the 9th day :-

Oestradiol valerate (Progynon depot)

Dose : 1ml. – I/M

- A heifer shows the heat symptoms after first injection (i.e. progynon depot 1 ml.) but she should not be inseminated. Again the heifer shows heat symptoms after receiving second dose of oestradiol valerate on 9th day. Inseminate the heifer or cow, 12 hours and 36 hours after the second injection of estradiol valerate.
- The development of udder is evident after one week onwards and from 15th day, onwards milk let down started gradually.
- This method induces fertile heat in heifer and also **induces lactation.**

If you point one big finger at someone, three fingers are pointing at you
– Edward Gibbon

Chapter 44

Hormonal Drugs Acting on the Reproductive System

The use of hormones is a major component of theriogenology. Hormonal preparations are utilized as reproductive managemental tools, diagnostic aids and therapeutic agents. In this chapter the main emphasis is given on the use of hormonal drugs for therepeutic management of reproductive disorders in cattle and buffalo.

Gonadotrophin-releasing Hormone (GnRH):

Gonadorelin and **Buserelin** are synthetic analogues of GnRH in which specific amino acid substitutions have been made in their molecular structure resulting in reduced susceptibility to proteolytic enzymes and greater affinity for binding to GnRH receptors. **Therefore GnRH analogue has about ten times potency than natural GnRH.**

Buserelin :

Pharmacological action :

Stimulate a short surge of FSH and LH following a single bolus injection which causes follicular development, oestrus and ovulation.

Indications :

Cattle

- Anoestrus - 20 µg (i.e 5 ml.), repeat after 8-22 days, if required.
- Delayed ovulation - 10µg (i.e 2.5 ml.) 6-8 hours before or at the time of insemination.
- Improvement of pregnancy rate - 2.5 ml. 6-8 hours before or at the time of insemination or **11-12 days after insemination.**
- Follicular cyst - 5ml, repeat after 10-14 days if required.

INTERESTING FACT
GnRH-induced LH release does not cause ovulation in oestrus mares, because normal preovulatory gonadotrophin surge occurs over a period of days, not in hours like a cow. Therefore, 40 mg (10 ml.) buserelin should be administered 6 hours before insemination and repeated after 1 day, if required. This example illustrates the importance of knowing the normal endocrine pattern in a given species when designing treatment or evaluating response to hormonal therapy.

Commercially available product :

Receptal (Intervet) 0.0042 mg/ml, 10 ml. vial.

Dose :
- Cattle – 10-20 µg (total dose)
- Horse – 40µg (total dose)

Route : Intramuscular (**preferred**) or intravenous.

Gonadorelin :

Indications and dose :
- Cystic ovaries – 500 µg, repeat if required.
- In conjunction with AI – 250 µg.
- Postpartum anoestrus – 500 µg repeat after 1-3 weeks.

Commercially available product :

Fertagyl (Intervet), 100 µg/ml, 1ml amp.

Cystorelin (BCAHP), 50 µg/ml. 2ml. & 10 ml. vial.

Route – Intramuscular.

Human Chorionic Gonadotrophin (hCG) :

It is a complex glycoprotein excreted in the urine of women during pregnancy. It has primarily similar effect to LH secreted by the anterior pituitary gland. Hence it is used as a substitute for the more expensive LH. It also has longer half-life than LH.

Pharmacological action :

hCG mimics the effect of LH causing ovulation. It promotes the formation and maintenance of corpus luteum in females.

Indications and dose :

Delayed ovulation or anovulation – 1500 IU-I/M at the time of A.I.

- Follicular cyst- 3000 IU-I/V.
- Repeat breeders – 1500 IU-I/M.

Commercially available product :

Chorulon (Intervet) 1500 IU vial

INTERESTING FACT
The major clinical advantage of hCG over pituitary LH (exogenous or GnRH-induced) is its long half-life, which increases its effectiveness for inducing ovulation in species like the mare, in which the normal LH surge is prolonged.

Pregnant Mare Serum Gonadotrophin (PMSG or eCG) :

It is also a complex glycoprotein. It is extracted from mare's serum during the *first trimester of pregnancy*. The effect of eCG is similar to FSH.

Pharmacological action :

It induces follicular growth in inactive ovaries of mature animals.

Indications :

Cattle :

- Superovulation.
- True anoestrus.

Commercially available products :

- *Folligon* (Intervet) 1000 IU vial + Solvent.

Dose and route :

1500-3000 IU – I/M or I/V.

Note : *In the treatments of anoestrus, AI should not be done in this induced oestrus.*

Hydroxy-progesterone Caproate :

Pharmacological action :

It mimics the action of corpus luteum.

Indications:
- Postpartum anoestrus
- Threatened abortion or habitual abortion
- Early embryonic death.

Dose and route :
- 500 mg intramuscular
- **Early habitual abortion** - 500 mg after 1.5 months of pregnancy, repeat at every 10 days.
- **Late habitual abortion** - 500 mg for 3 days followed by 500 mg/week.

Commercially available products :
- *Duraprogen* (Vetcare) 250 mg/ml, 2ml. amp.
- *P-depot* (Sarabhai-Zydus) 250 mg/ml, 2ml. amp.

Oestrogen :

Pharmacological action :

Oestrogen is primarily responsible for oestrus behaviour in the female. It increases the natural defence mechanism against infection. Therefore, oestrogen is used to treat chronic endometritis. *It must not be used in acute uterine infections because it enhances the absorption of bacterial toxins.* Oestrogen is used in the treatment of misalliance in the bitch. It acts by inhibiting the transport of the fertilized ova from the oviduct to the uterus.

Oestrogen is also called epitheliotropic hormone, since vasostimulation and general health of the skin are favoured. This is why the female has a softer, thinner, and more luxuriant skin than the male.

Side-effect : *Over dose may cause severe inhibition of pituitary function and cystic ovaries in cattle and pigs.*

Indications
- Ripening of cervix in case of dystocia
- Chronic endometritis
- Pyometra
- Mummification
- Hydramnios and hydrallantois.

Commercially available products

Progynon depot (Oestradiol valerate) 10mg/ml, 1ml amp.

Dose : 5-10 mg/ml., repeat at 7-days intervals, if required.

Prostaglandins :

- **Cloprostenol, dinoprost, luprostiol and tiaprost** are synthetic $PGF_2\alpha$ or analogues available for use in veterinary practice.
- *The corpus luteum is refractory (resistant) to the action of $PGF_2\alpha$ analogues for at least 5 days after ovulation in mares, cows, ewes and does while in sows, the refractory period is up to 11 days.*
- In bitches and queens, the CL is generally unresponsive at any time after ovulation unless subjected to repeated doses.
- The primary effect of $PGF2\alpha$ on the reproductive system is regression of corpus luteum.

Indications :

- Pyometra
- Mummification
- Endometritis
- Luteal cyst
- Induction of parturition
- Synchronisation of oestrus
- Silent heat.

WARNING
<ul><li>$PGF_2\alpha$ can be absorbed through the skin and may cause bronchospasm or miscarriage (abortion). Therefore care should be taken when handling the product to avoid self-injection or skin contact.</li><li>Women of child-bearing age, asthmatics, and persons with bronchial or other respiratory problems should avoid to contact or wear disposable gloves while administering the product.</li><li>Accidental spillage on the skin should be washed off immediately with soap and water.</li><li>In the event of accidental·administration to a person, medical advice should be sought promptly.</li></ul>

Commercially available products and their doses

Cloprostenol :
  Vetmate (Vetcare) 2 ml. vial
  Synchromate (Prima vetcare) 2 ml. vial
  Dose - 2 ml. I/M.

Dinoprost
  Lutalyse (Novartis) 5 mg/ml, 10 ml. vial
  Dose - 25 mg or 5 ml. I/M.

Luprostiol
  Prosolvin (Intervet) 7.5 mg/ml, 2ml. vial
  Dose - Cow-15 mg. or 2 ml I/M
  Heifer & mare - 7.5 mg. or 1 ml. I/M

Tiaprost :
  Iliren (Intervet) 0.196 mg/ml ,10 ml vial
  Dose - 3.5 ml I/Vor 5ml I/M

Myometrial stimulant - Oxytocin :

- Oxytocin stimulates contraction of the *oestrogen-sensitized myometrium*. This activity may be of benefit in dystocia due to secondary uterine inertia.
- Oxytocin should not be used when dystocia is related to malposition or malpresentation or foeto-maternal disproportion.
- Many recommended dose rates are too high. The myometrium is very sensitive to the effects of oxytocin and high dose rate causes spasms rather than synchronized contractions.
- Oxytocin is most effective when used in an intravenous drip in saline.
- Oxytocin must be used within 12 hours of calving, after which myometrial sensitivity to its action is reduced.
- Oxytocin has been recommended to evacuate the udder of the cow in the treatment of mastitis.
- Oxytocin injections are recommended to induce contractions of the uterus after caesarean section.

Indications :

- Postpartum haemorrhage

- Retention of placenta
- Primary uterine inertia
- Uterine involution after dystocia
- Prolapse of uterus (After replacement)
- Agalactia due to failure of milk let-down.

Commercially available products :

Oxytocin (Local) 5 IU/ml,1 ml amp.

Pitocin (Parke-Davis)   5 IU/0.5 ml,0.5 ml. amp.

Syntocinon (Novartis pharma) 5 IU/ml,1 ml. amp.

Dose :

	Obstetrics	Milk let down
Mare –	75 – 150 IU	10 – 20 IU
Cow –	75 – 100 IU	10 – 20 IU
Sow –	30 – 50 IU	5 – 20 IU
Ewe –	30-50 IU	5 – 20 IU
Bitch –	5-25 IU	2 – 10 IU
Queen –	5-10 IU	1 – 10 IU

Precaution : *Administration of oxytocin in dystocia, without sufficient cervical dilatation, is contra-indicated.*

Myometrial Relaxants :

- These drugs cause **relaxation** of the uterus and are used to aid in **obstetrical correction** during dystocia and to facilitate handling of the uterus during **caesarean section**.
- These drugs are also used to facilitate replacement of a **prolapsed uterus**.
- They can be used to **delay parturition during night** so that greater observation and care are available during day time.
- They are used in heifers, so that **calving can be delayed sufficiently** to allow better relaxation of the birth canal and perineum.

Pharmacological action :

- **Clenbuterol** and **isoxsuprine** are **beta-adrenergic agents**. The smooth muscles of the uterus contain β_2- **adrenergic receptors**, which when stimulated, cause relaxation of myometrium and abolition of uterine contractions. Clenbuterol is a highly selective and long-acting stimulator of β_2-adrenergic receptors.

- *These drugs cause easy parturition because dilatation of the cervix and softening of the birth canal continue during the period of tocolysis.*

- A beneficial effect of clenbuterol in cases of dystocia is an improvement in the supply of blood to the placenta and foetus (mediated by β_2 vasodilation of blood vessels). *Therefore, viability of calves is unimpaired and subsequent fertility is normal.*

- *The tocolytic effect of clenbuterol can be reversed by the administration of oxytocin and prostaglandins.*

- Once the tocolytic effect of clenbuterol wears off, normal parturition resumes. No adverse effects are seen and parturition are shortened and easier than usual, especially in heifers.

Indications :
- Dystocia
- Foetotomy
- Caesarean section
- Prolapse of uterus
- Parturition in night
- Parturition in heifers.

Dose and route :
- Clenbuterol (trade name *Planipart* 30 µg/ml).

  Cattle – 0.3 mg or 10 ml (total dose) I/M or slow I/V or 60 µg/ 100 kg. b.w.

- Isoxsuprine (trade name *Duvadilan/Suprox* 5 mg/ml, 2 ml. amp) Cattle – 115-230 mg (total dose)

CLINICAL POINTER

Mix 4 to 10 ampoules of Duvadilan in 500 ml. water and apply locally on the prolapsed mass of uterus with the help of cotton. It makes the prolapsed mass soft and becomes easy to push inside.

Night and Clenbuterol
• Clenbuterol is specifically used to **postpone parturition** in cattle at the night as a managemental aid. For this, it is given at a dose rate of 0.3 mg (**10 ml**) intramuscularly at about 6 PM followed by a second injection of 0.21 mg (**7ml**) at 10 PM. This protocol postpones calving for 8 hours after the second injection.
• It should always be remembered that if the cervix is fully dilated, it (Clenbuterol) must not be used.

Valethamide Bromide :

Pharmacological action :

It is a quaternary ammonium compound, with peripheral actions similar to those of atropine enabling cervical dilatation.

Indications :

• Inadequate cervical dilatation at the time of parturition.
• Kinked cervix.

Dose :

Cattle and mare	-	40-50 mg I/M
Sheep, goat and pig	-	10-20 mg I/M
Dog and cat	-	5-10 mg I/M

Market preparations :

• *Epidosin vet* (10 mg/ml) 10 ml. vial
• *Epidosin* (8 mg/ml) 1ml ampoule

Clomiphene Citrate :

Pharmacological action :

Clomiphene inhibits negative feedback mechanism of oestrogen on GnRH, enabling the release of GnRH from hypothalamus, inducing the ovulation.

Indications :

• Anovulatory oestrus
• Repeat breeding
• Delayed puberty

- Anoestrus
- Silent heat
- Delayed ovulation.

Dose :

Cattle, horse, sheep, goat and pig- 1-1.5 mg/kg. b.w. for 5 days orally.

Dog – 25 mg/kg b.w. orally.

Mode of administration : One tablet should be dissolved in 500 ml of water. Just before drenching the medicine, 125 ml 10% sodium bicarbonate or 1% copper sulphate should be drenched which closes the reticular groove so that the medicine goes to the abomasum directly.

Market preparations :

- *Fertivet* 300 mg. tab.
- *Clofert* 25 mg., 50 mg. and 100 mg. tab.
- *Clofert vet* 300 mg. tab.

Reticular Groove Reflex :

For proper rumen development in the suckling animal, it is important for milk to be diverted away from the developing rumen. This is accomplished by the actions of the reticular groove (also called the oesophageal groove). Reticular groove is a **gutter-like invagination** traversing the wall of the reticulum from the **cardia to the reticulo-omasal orifice**. Reticular groove closure is a reflex action with efferent impulses arriving from the brainstem through the vagus nerve. Afferent stimuli arise centrally and from the pharynx. Fluid especially sodium-containing fluid in the pharynx stimulates the reflex action. When stimulated, muscles of the groove contract causing it to shorten and twist. The twisting action causes the lips of the groove to close together, forming a nearly complete tube from the cardia to the omasal canal. Milk entering the cardia when groove is contracted is directed into the omasum. Milk quickly traverses the omasum and enters the abomasum. The reticular groove has its primary function in suckling animals, and the activity of the groove reflex appears to **diminish after weaning and with advancing age.**

CLINICAL IMPORTANCE OF RETICULAR GROOVE REFLEX

- Beneficial uses of the reticular groove reflex have been neglected in practical veterinary medicine.

- Oral administration of drugs intended for local intestinal effect (i.e. purgative, antidiarrhoeals and some anthelmintics) should always be preceded by administration of an appropriate salt solution to close the groove.

- In cattle, closure of the groove can be elicited with 10% sodium bicarbonate or sodium sulphate, whereas in sheep 5% copper sulphate is effective.

- Closure of the groove takes about 2-5 seconds and it often remains **closed for up to 60 seconds.**

❈ ❈ ❈ ❈ ❈

Talk to yourself positively all the time : "I feel happy ! I feel healthy ! I feel successful !

Chapter 45

Homoeopathy in Female Reproductive Disorders

The use of homoeopathy represents an entirely different philosophy from that of conventional medicine. Veterinary homoeopathy has a tradition almost as long as homoeopathy for humans. Veterinary homoepathy is at least 180 years old. Homoeopathic treatment of animals was introduced by **Baron Von Boenninghausen**. Von Boenninghausen treated various species of animals and is said to have established the principle of veterinary homoeopathy. Veterinary homöeopathy has its strongest modern tradition in Europe, particularly in Germany, France and Great Britain. In the united states the Academy of Veterinary Homoeopathy offers a course in veterinary classic homoeopathy. In India, many veterinarians are treating the animal with homoepathic medicine. Homoeopathic treatment is cost effective also.

Administration of homoeopathic medicines :

- In all cases, when possible the medicines should be given to animals when they have been for sometime without food, say **15-30 minutes before they are fed.**

- As a general rule, the usual potencies (strength of the drug) selected for animals are tincture (Q), 30, 200 and 1000.

- Repeatation of doses : This is a matter which must depend entirely upon the severity of the disease. In **per acute cases,** the dose may be **given every ten, fifteen or thirty minutes; in acute cases, every two, three or four hours; in chronic cases, once or twice daily.**

- 5 – 10 drops of the appropriate potency of medicine should be placed on the tongue of the animal or mixed with a morsel of any favourite article of food.

- To make the lotion of arnica, calendula or Rhus tox, mix one table–spoonful of the tincture (Q) with **half a pint** (1 pint = 473 ml.) **of pure water.** The lotion is applied on the affected parts, twice or thrice daily.

Vesicular vaginitis :

- **Cantharis 30** – Frequent urination with straining and vesicular inflammation of the genital tract call for this remedy.

  Dose : 5 - 10 drops three times daily for five days.

- **Hydrastis 30** – This is a very good remedy for **any catarrhal condition** arising as a result of inflammation affecting **mucus membrane.** It is therefore applicable to uterine conditions discharging muco-purulent materials.

  Dose : 5-10 drops three times daily for five days.

Abortion :

It has frequent occurrence among cows. When abortion threatens, it is generally indicated by premonitory symptoms. By using appropriate homoeopathic drugs, it can be prevented.

- **Arnica 30/200 :** If during gestation, an animal is known to have received an injury, it is advisable to administer this remedy at once and repeat it as often as the nature of the case seems to require. If promptly given, it will prevent miscarriage under such circumstances.

  Dose : 5-10 drops three-four times daily for 4-5 days.

- **Rhus tox : 30/200** if miscarriage is threatened in consequence of strains over extension, administer this remedy instead of arnica.

  Dose : 5-10 drops three-four times daily for 4-5 days.

- **Secale 30 :** If the symptoms of abortion have actually set in, this remedy will facilitate labour. It is **called for violent straining** after abortion and abundant discharge of blood.

  Dose : 5-10 drops every two hours for four doses.

- **Pulsatilla 30 :** This will sometimes avert abortion by lessening uterine pains.

  Dose : 5-10 drops every two or three hours till symptoms subside.

- **Viburnum opulus 200 :** To rule out any specific cause of abortion and to prevent abortion.

  Dose : 5-10 drops three times daily for 7 days and then repeat weekly.

Puerperal metritis :

- **Aconitum Napellus 6** : It is particularly indicated in those cases which arise with sudden intensity. It helps in **reducing shock and fears.**

  Dose : 5-10 drops every half-hour for six doses.

- **Belladona 1M** : A useful remedy when there is a **full bounding pulse, hot skin** and **dilated pupils** with signs of impending delirium.

  Dose - 5-10 drops three-four times daily.

- **Echinacea 3X** : Indicated where **systemic involvement** is rapid and signs of **septicaemia** are present. Temperature remains high and respirations are shallow. This is a remedy which acts **best in lower potencies.**

  Dose : 5-10 drops every two hours for four doses.

- **Sabina 6** : This a is useful remedy when puerperal metritis is associated with retention of placenta. This is a useful remedy for **controlling blood stained discharges.**

  Dose : 5-10 drops every two hours for four doses.

- **Secale 30 :** This is indicated in somewhat similar picture to sabina, but discharges **contain dark fluid blood** and the animal has a **lean or cadaverous appearance.** Signs of disturbance to the peripheral circulation may be present; for example, **cold extremities and lack of sensation.**

  Dose : 5-10 drops three times daily for four days.

Suboestrus or silent heat :

- **Sepia 200** : It should be given as a routine remedy because it has generally **tonic effect on ovaries and uterus.**

  Dose : 5-10 drops once only (single dose).

- **Pulsatilla 200** : It is a **very good ovarian remedy** sometimes associated with vaginal discharge of a creamy consistency.

  Dose : 5-10 drops per alternate day for three weeks.

- **Platina 6** : It has beneficial action on ovarian function.

  Dose : 5-10 drops daily for one week.

Retention of placenta :

- Sepia 1M + Sabina 200 : 5-10 drops hourly (per hours) for five hours. **or**

- Cantharis – 5-10 drops hourly for five hours **or**
- Caulophylum 200 + Pyrogenium 200 + Secale cornutum 30 : 5-10 drops hourly for five hours **or**
- Gossypum mother tincture : One tea spoonful once in three hours interval till foetal membranes fall off.

  After removal of retained foetal membranes
- Sepia 1M + Caulophyllum 200

  Dose – 5-10 drops three times daily for 3 days.
- If RFM has occurred 24 hours earlier, then ½ ml of **Apis mellifica CM** potency is used as **subcutaneous injection.**
- Pulsatilla 30 : It is also useful in the treatment of RFM.

True anoestrus :

- **Pulsatilla 30** : Should be given in silent heat.
- **Calcarea phosphorica 30. Dose** – 5-10 drops for three days, followed by one dose every second day for three doses.
- **Iodum 30** : This is a good remedy if the **ovaries are felt small and shrivelled** on rectal examination. Suitable for **lean animals with good appetite and active temperament.**

  Dose : 5-10 drops daily for ten days.

Cystic ovaries :

- **Apis mellifica 6** : This is a useful remedy for dissolving cysts by causing absorption of fluid.

  Dose : 5-10 drops daily for three weeks.
- **Murex purpurea 30** : A good **remedy for nymphomania** and for regulating the oestrous cycle.

  Dose : 5-10 drops per week for three weeks.
- **Platina 30** : A very **good ovarian remedy** in general.

  Dose : 5-10 drops three times daily for five days.
- **Palladium 6** : If the **right ovary alone** is affected this remedy could well be indicated.

  Dose : 5-10 drops twice daily for one week.
- **Oopherinium 6X** : This ovarian extract frequently brings about resolution of the cyst, if used in low potency.

  Dose – 5-10 drops daily for five days.

Persistent corpus luteum (Pyometra, mummification) :

- **Folliculinim 6 :**
  Dose : 5-10 drops daily for 5 days.
- **Pulsatilla 30 :** It acts on the ovarian tissues and helpls to restore normal ovary function.
  Dose : 5-10 drops daily for 5 days.
- **Sepia 200C : It regulates the activity of the genital tract and is aiding the action of other remedies.**
  Dose : 5-10 drops as a single dose.
- **Thuja 6 :** If CL is in **left ovaries.**

Anovulatory heat :

- **Sepia 200** – 5-10 drops as a single dose.
- **Pulsatilla 30** – There may be an accompanying vaginal discharge of semi-purulent material.
  Dose : 5-10 drops per week for three weeks.
- **Calcarea phosphorica 30 :** Useful remedy for yonger animals (heifers). If **catarrhal vaginal discharge** is present, then also it is indicated.
  Dose : 5-10 drops per week for three weeks.
- **Iodum 30** – It is indicated when **smooth ovaries** are present.
  Dose : 5-10 drops daily for 10 days.
- **Oopherinium 6X :** The ovarian extract may be **used in conjunction with other remedies.**
  Dose : 5-10 drops daily for five days.

Dystocia :

- **Arnica 30 :** 5-10 drops at 2 hours' intervals for four doses.
- **Pulsatilla 30 :** 5-10 drops once.

Prepartum prolapse of vagina :

After replacing the prolapsed mass, following drugs can be tried :
- **Murex 6/30 :** 5-10 drops twice a weeks for 4 to 6 weeks.
- **Calcaria phos 30 :** It is given to remove deficiency of calcium & phosphorus.
  Dose : 5-10 drops twice a day for 10 days, then thrice a week till parturition.

- **Arnica 30** : 5-10 drops four times daily.

Post-partum prolapse of uterus :

After replacing the prolapsed mass, following drugs can be tried.
- **Aloes 30** : 5-10 drops thrice a day for a week.
- **Sepia 30** : In acute case, 5-10 dropes four times a day.
- **Calcaria phos 30 + Cal. Carb 30**

  Dose : 5-10 drops thrice a day for a week.

Repeat breeders :

Start treatment immediately after the end of oestrum with **sepia 200** 5 drops TID for one day allow three days gap, start **Aurum iodum 200 and Thyroidinum 30,** each drug is given 5-10 drops 3 times a day for 10 days, allow two days gap and give **Agnus castus 200,** 5 to 10 drops TID till the next oestrum is noticed. Aurum iodum and Thyroidinum have a role in improving the relationship between **ovary and thyroid gland.** If **milk yield drops,** Thyroidinum should be discontinued.

Incomplete dilatation of cervix or failure of cervical dilatation:

Caulophyllum 200 : 5-10 drops once in 15 minutes interval can be given if **presentation, position and posture are normal.**

Commonly used homoeopathic drugs in injury :

Hypericum :   Injury to areas rich in nerve ending (eg. digit, tail etc.), injury to nerves, photosensitization.

Ledum :   Punctured wound.

Aconitum :   Sudden shock to the mind or body. Sudden disturbances of the body's equilibrium (eg. sudden – onset fever, **sudden haemorrhage).**

Calendula :   Open wound; acts as antiseptic and promotes healing.

Arnica :C   losed wound.

Organ-specific homoeopathic remedies :

Rhus tox :   Muscles

Ruta graveolens : Tendons, ligaments & joint capsules.

Hypericum :   Nerve fibres.

Symphytum : Bone
Nux vomica : Liver
Lycopodium : Liver
Berberis : Liver, kidney
Kali chloratum: Kidney
Digitalis : Heart

Common homoeopathic drugs and their uses :

Name of drugs	Uses

Aconitum napellus :
* Acute cases
* Shock
* Sudden–onset of fever
* Disorders from chilling and cold winds.

Allium cepa :
* Profuse nasal discharge (typical coryza).

Apis mellifica :
* **Insect (bee) bites**
* Oedema and swelling anywhere.
* Pulmonary oedema.
* Oedamatous swelling of vulvar perineum or udder
* Ascites
* Cystic ovaries.

Arnica montana :
* Used in all conditions arising from trauma.
* **Used in the wounds where the skin remains unbroken.**
* Marked affinity with blood vessels.
* Prevent haemorrhage.
* **During pregnancy prevent threatened abortion due to mechanical injuries from blows or falls.**

313

Arsenicum album :	* Profuse, watery and offensive smelling diarrhoea.
Aurum muriaticum natro natrum :	* Fibrosed udder.
Belladonna :	* Antinflammatory.
	* Analgesic.
	* Antipyretic
	* Acute mastitis
Borax :	* Vesicular stomatitis and allied diseases.
	* **For prevention of FMD diseases.**
Bryonia :	* Act on **serous membranes.**
	* Affected animal is unwilling to move.
	* Pneumonia
	* Mastitis
	* Arthritis
	* Peritonitis
Calendula :	* Used for local application in open wound
	* Helps in healing wounds by fast granulation tissue formation.
Carbo vegetabilis :	* Ruminal stasis
	* **Bloat**
	* Cold
	* This remedy is called **homoeopathic corpse (dead body) reviver.** So it is used in collapsed individual.
Caulophyllum:	* All disorders of parturition at any stage.
	* **Revive labour pains.**
	* **Can be used as alternative to oxytocin**

* Uterine torsion.
* Retention of placenta
* Cervical dilatation if presentation, position and posture of foetus is normal.

Colocynthis :
* Colic
* To alleviate acute bloat **with lycopodium.**

Dulcamara :
* Remedy for all those conditions which arise as a result of **exposure to wet and cold,** especially when damp evening follows a warm day.
* Helpful for let down of milk in cold season.

Hepar sulphuris :
* **If any homoeopathic remedy could be said to fill the** role of antibiotics in septic conditions, then this is the one.
* Abscess which is **extremely sensitive to touch.**
* Mastitis
* Low potency – Promote suppuration.
* High potency (200 and upwards) – abort the purulent process.

Glonoinum :
* **Heat stroke.**

Hecla lava :
* Actinomycosis

Hydrastis :
* Mild form of metritis.

Hypericum perforatum :
* Injury to nerves or to areas rich in nerve endings.
* Photosensitization

Ipecacuana :
* Postpartum bleeding.
* Blood in milk.
* Coccidiosis in calves.

Murex purpurea :

* Anoestrus
* Delayed ovulation.
* Anovulator heat.
* Folliculary cyst.

Nux vomica :

* Digestive disturbances
* Ruminal stasis
* Labour pain
* Appetizer
* **Nullifies the bad effects of many homoepathic drugs and allopathic drugs**

Palladium :

* Ovarian dysfunctions.

Pulsatilla :

* Ovarian hypofunction.
* Retained placenta.

Phytolacca :

* Mastitis (when milk becomes thickened, stringy and yellowish).

Rhus toxicodendron :

* Muscle injury.
* Sprain

Ruta graveolens :

* Injury to tendons, ligaments and joint capsules.
* Sprains.
* **Facilitate labour by increasing the tone of uterine** contractions.

Sabina :

* **Postpartum fresh bleeding.**
* Retained foetal membranes.

Secale :

* Post partum **dark coloured bleeding.**

Sepia :

* Regulate the entire oestrous cycle.
* **Should always be given as a routine preliminary remedy in gynaecological discords.**
* Post partum infections.

	* Capable of encouraging the **natural maternal instinct in** those animals which do not allow the calf to suck the milk.
Silicea :	* Chronic abscess.
	* Summer mastitis.
	* **Stimulate expulsion of foreign bodies from the tissues.**
Sulphur :	* **Inter-current remedy to aid the action of other** remedies.
	* Mange and eczema.
	* **Impure milk.**
Thuja :	* Warty growth which bleeds easily.
	* Papillomatous warts.
	* Ill effect of vaccination.

Any good that you can do, do it now. Do not delay it, for you will not pass this way again.

Chapter 46

Drugs Commonly Used in Bovine Reproductive Disorders

Generic names	Trade names	Indications	Dose and route
1. GnRH analogues :			
(a) Buserelin	Receptal (10ml. vial)	* Anoestrus * Silent oestrus * Follicular cyst * Anovulation *Delayed ovulation * Improvement of conception rate.	5ml. IM 2.5 ml. IM at the time of AI.
(b) Gonadorelin	* Fertagyl * Cystorelin	- do -	5 ml. IM
2. hCG	Chorulon	- do -	1500-3000 IU-IM
3. PMSG	Folligon (1000 IU/ vial)	* True anoestrus * Superovulation	1500-3000 IU-IM/IV
4. Hydroxy progesterone caproate (250 mg/ml.)	Duraprogen (2 ml. amp)	* Theartened abortion * Habitual abortion * Eary embryonic death	500 mg. IM
5. PGF₂α analogues			
a. Cloprostenol	Vetmate (2 ml. vial)	* Luteal cyst * Mummification * Pyometra * Silent oestrus * Induction of parturition	2 ml. IM.
b. Dinoprost (5 mg/ml)	Lutalyse (5 ml vial)	- do -	5ml. IM
c. Luprostiol (7.5 mg./ml)	Prosolvin (2 ml. amp.)	- do -	2ml. IM
d. Tiaprost	Iliren (10 ml. vial)	- do -	5ml. IM,IV,SC

Drugs Commonly Used in Bovine Reproductive Disorders

Generic names	Trade names	Indications	Dose and route
6. Oestradiol valerate (10 mg/ml)	Progynon depot	* Mummification * Maceration * Pyometra * Uterine inertia * Uterine infection	3-10 mg. IM
7. Oxytocin (5 units/ml.)	Pitocin (1ml. amp)	* Uterine inertia * Dystocia * Retention of placenta * Uterine prolapse	75-50 IU, IM, IV
8. Ergometrine (0.5 mg/ml.)	Ergometrine (1ml. amp)	Post partum bleeding	1-3 mg. IM
9. Isoxsuprine (5mg/ml)	Duvadilan (2ml amp)	Uterine prolapse	0.5 mg/kg IM
10. V alethamide bromide (10mg./ml)	Epidosin vet 10 ml., 30ml. vial	* Inadequate cervical dilatation during parturition	40-50 mg IM
11. Clomiphene	Fertivet (300 mg tab)	* Anovulatory oestrus * Repeat breeders	300 mg orally for 5 days
12. Vit. A (3 lakh IU/ml)	* Prepalin forte (2ml.) * Vit. A (2ml.)	Infertility	12ml. /week IM
13. Vitamin AD₃ E	* Vetade (5ml) * Vitacept (5ml) * Vitamin AD₃E * Intavita	- do -	2 vial/week IM
14. Vit. E and selenium	E-care-se (10ml)	- do -	1ml/25-50kg IM
15. Vitamin K (100mg/ml)	Kaplin (1ml.)	Haemorrhage	0.5-2ml/100kg IM/IV
16. Vitamin C	Ascorbic acid (5ml)	Infertility	15-20ml/100kg. IV
17. Iron (50 mg/ml)	Imferon (10ml.)	Haemorrhage	5-10ml. – IM
18. Phosphorus	* Tonophosphon (30ml) * Urimin (30 ml)	Anoestrus	10ml. IM alternate day for three days.
19. Calcium borogluconate	* Calboral (450 ml) * Intacal (450 ml)	* Uterine inertia * Milk fever	400-800ml IV
20. Calcium and magnesium borogluconate	* Mifex (450 ml) * Lactomag (450 ml)	- do -	- do -

Generic names	Trade names	Indications	Dose and route
21. Adr enaline (1mg/ml)	Adrenaline (1 ml)	Haemorrhage	* 8-16ml/100kg IM * 4-8ml/100kg IV * Apply locally
22. Car bazochrome	* Starden (10ml,30ml) * Chromstate (10ml, 30ml) * Adchrome (10ml,30ml)	Haemorrhage	10ml IM
Intrauterine preparations :			
23. Cip rofloxacin & Tinidazole	C-Flox-TZ suspension (60 ml)	Uterine infection	60 ml. I/U repeat for 3-5 days.
24. Cep halexin dry susp.	Lixen IU (4.5gm)	- do -	4.5 gm I/U for 3-5 days. Dissolve the contents of vial in 60 ml. distilled water.
25. Oxy tetracycline	* Steclin bolus * Oxytetracyclin powder	- do -	2-4 boli I/U 1-2 gm I/U
26. Nitr ofurazone and urea	Furea	- do -	2 – 4 boli I/U
27. Nitr ofurazone, metronidazole and urea	* Pesurea * Uterofit * Utex	- do -	2 – 4 boli I/U
28. Nitr ofurazone, metronidazole & povidone iodine	* Cleanex	- do -	2 – 4 boli I/U
29. Pov idone iodine (5% w/v)	Wokadine (100ml)	- do -	10 – 40 ml I/U
30. Pov idone iodine and metronidazole metronidazole	Ranvidone I.U. (60ml)	- do -	30 – 60 ml. I/U

Herbal drugs :

Herbal drugs	Indications	Dose and route
31. Involon (500 ml, 1 litre & 5 litres)	**In freshly calved animals** * To prevent retention of placenta. * For timely involution of uterine horns. * As uterine tonic and cleansing agent. **In cases of retained placenta** * To facilitate easy expulsion of retained placenta. * To assist in manual removal.	Loading dose of 200ml on first day followed by 100ml. for 3 consecutive days.
32. Uterotone liquid	- do -	- do -
33. Utrifit	- do -	- do -
34. Replanta (500gm & 1kg)	- do -	Initial dose 100 gm. followed by 50-60 gm. QID.
35. Prolapse - in	Vaginal and uterine prolapse	5 tabs BID orally for 4-5 days.
36. Prajana HS	Anoestrus	3 caps/day for 2 days. Repeat on 11th and 12th day, in case of no oestrus signs.
37. Sajani	- do -	- do -
38. Janova	- do -	- do -
39. Myron	* Uterine infection * Cervicitis * Vaginitis * Atonic reproductive tract	10 tab BID orally for 2-3 weeks.
40. Leptaden vet	Galactogogue	10 tab BID orally for 2 weeks.

Minerals mixtures preparations :

Minerals	Indications	Dose and route
41. Chelated agrimin forte (1kg, 2 kg and 5 kg)	To improve breeding efficiency	25-30 gm. orally for one month.
42. Minal forte	- do -	- do -
43. Metho-chelated bestmin gold	- do -	- do -
44. Minfa	- do -	- do -
45. COFECU plus	- do -	1 tab daily
46. Cyclomin-7 bolus	- do -	1 bolus/week
47. Minotas bolus	- do -	2 bolus daily for 2 weeks.

321

Chelated minerals :

- Now-a-days, in the market, different pharmaceutical companies are launching chelated mineral mixture. Hence, it is essential for the students and clinicians to know about the chelated minerals.

- **Chelated minerals : "The chelation process involves the chemical bonding of the trace minerals to an amino acid(s) or small peptides."** Chelated minerals is a way of presenting the essential trace minerals to the cow in a form that is more readily absorbed and utilized and not subject to the same interactions commonly experienced with inorganic elemental forms.

The advantage of *in vitro* Mineral Chelation :

Chelation enhances bioabsorption because the organic form is recognized as peptide or amino acid.

Chelation protects mineral in adverse medium.

Chelation protects minerals' from incompatibility situation in presence of antagonistic element (s).

Chelation makes minerals pH stable and electrically neutral.

Chelation improves tissue mineral retention and activity.

Chelation makes specific tissue target of minerals e.g., If Zinc is chelated with methionine, it will be targeted to hooves, skin, epithelial tissue regeneration and hair, where it is needed in large quantities.

Chelation is proven to be beneficial in situations like reproductive problems, stress and rations with various interfering substances such as phytin, where ordinary trace minerals supplementation fails.

Adding essential trace minerals in chelated form is a proven useful means for solving several practical problems.

Infertility :

- The process of pregnancy is dependent on essential trace minerals, which influence immune system, hormonal patterns and the integrity of regenerated cellular epithelium.

- The latest evidences also suggest that originally bound trace minerals may have a beneficial role to play in the resumption of follicular growth and fertility in dairy cows.

- The trials with chelated minerals' supplementation during the first 100 days following parturition has been shown to increase fertility in dairy cows through increased conception rate and improved embryonic survival.

The improved reproduction by chelated mineral supplementation results from :

- Reduced embryonic death loss.
- Improved uterine environment.
- Reduced incidence of cystic ovaries.
- Increased intensity of oestrous behaviour.

Calculation of Drug Doses :

How to calculate milliliters (ml) needed :

Total dose needed (mg) = Dose (mg/kg) x body weight of animal (kg)

Strength of solution (mg/ml) = (% strength) x 10

$$\text{ml needed} = \frac{\text{Total dose needed}}{\text{Strength of solution (mg/ml)}}$$

Example : 300 kg. cow needs 5 mg/kg of a 10% w/v enrofloxacin injection.

Total dose needed = 5 x 300 mg. = 1500 mg.

Strength of solution (mg/ml) = 10 x 10 = 100

ml. needed = 1500/100 = 15 ml.

How to calculate tablets / boli needed

Total dose needed (mg) = Dose (mg/kg) x body weight of animal (kg)

$$\text{Number of tablet/bolus needed} = \frac{\text{Total dose needed}}{\text{Strength of tablet/bolus}}$$

Example :

20 kg. dog needs 12 mg/kg of a drug.

Tablet size is 100mg.

Total dose needed (mg) = 20 kg. x 12 mg/kg. = 240 mg.

Number of tablets needed = 240mg./100mg. = 2.4 tablets.

(In most instances, it is rounded up to 2.5 tablets if the medication has sufficient safety).

Common Prescription Writing Errors

- Always use metric units : e.g., **g** (gram) for solids; **ml** (milliliter) for liquids.
- Use **per** instead of a slash (/), which can be interpreted as the number **1**.
- Use **units** instead of the abbreviation **u** which can be interpreted as **0** or **4** or **m**.
- Use **once daily** instead of **sid**, which has been interpreted as **5 / d** or **5 per day**.

  (NOTE : "Sid" is not a conventional prescription abbreviation).
- Use **three times daily** instead of **tid**, and **four times daily** instead of **qid**.
- Use **every other day** instead of **qod**.
- REMEMBER – abbreviations like **qd, qid** and **qod** are easily confused with each other.
- When writing numbers :

  Use a **leading zero** with decimals : e.g., use **0.5 ml.** rather than **.5 ml.**

  Avoid using a trailing zero : e.g., use 3 rather than 3.0.
- And FINALLY – When in doubt .... spell it out.

❈ ❈ ❈ ❈ ❈

Thinking is the hardest work there is, which is the probable reason why so few engage in it **- Henry Ford.**

GLOSSARY

Special features :

- It covers almost all the commonly used **terminology** in veterinary gynaecology and obstetrics.
- It also covers few terminology from **human gynaecology**.
- It saves the valuable time as well as energy of students during preparation of examinations and interviews.
- It is arranged in **topic-wise** not in alphabetical order for easy rememembring of all the related terms.

GLOSSARY

Gynaecology: (From Greek, gynae means woman and logos means discourse or study). It pertains to the diseases of the female, but the term is generally used for diseases related to the female genital organs. "A branch of science which deals with the study of physio-pathology of reproduction, infective and non-infective conditions of genital tract affecting efficiency of reproduction is called Gynaecology".

Theriogenology : (Greek word 'therio = animal or beast and gen = coming into). The branch of science which deals with all aspects of veterinary obstetrics, genital diseases and animal reproduction, is called theriogenology. The term was first proposed by **D. Bartlett** and others.

Reproduction: "Reproduction is the ability of all living organisms to produce young ones similar to themselves in most of the characters". Reproduction is a luxury function of the body not physiologically necessary for life of the individual and usually not performed until the animal reaches nearly to adult size.

Obstetrics: (Latin word means 'midwife'). The branch of science which deals with the care of female during **gestation, parturition** and **puerperium** is called obstetrics.

Andrology: The branch of science which deals with the investigation and problems of infertility in male animals is called andrology.

Paediatrics: The branch of science that deals with the care of newborn in most critical stage of life when it is exposed to various external stimuli is called paediatrics.

Uniparous or Monotocous animal: The animal in which only one ovum is released at each ovulation and one foetus develop in the uterus is called uniparous or monotocous animal. The uniparous group of animals are characterized by the presence of a well developed cervix eg., cow, buffalo and mare.

Multiparous or polytocous animal: The animal in which more than one ova are released at ovulation and more than one foetus develop in the uterus, is called polytocous animal. In general, multiparous animals have a poorly developed cervix. eg., bitch, cat and sow.

Nullipara: Females that never conceived or carried young are called nullipara.

Primipara: Females that have conceived and have had only one gestation period are called primipara.

Pluripara: Females that have conceived two or more times and have had two or more gestation periods are called pluripara.

Puberty: It is the period when a male or female is first able to release gametes. In case of female, the first oestrus is the visible sign for attainment of puberty.

Fertility: Ability of an animal to reproduce maximum within the stipulated time as per the norms of the species is called fertility.

Infertility: Temporary inability of the animal to reproduce is called infertility.

Sub-fertility: Less than normal reproductive capacity is called subfertility.

Sterility: Permanent inability of an animal to reproduce is called sterility.

Adolescent sterility : Full reproductive efficiency is not attained in any species at the first oestrus or ejaculation. This is a period of adolescent sterility. This period is remarkably short (some weeks) in domestic animals as compared with humans (1 year or more).

Oestrous cycle: It is a chain of physiological events that begins at one oestrous period and ends at the next or it is a cycle of reproductive activity exhibited by sexually mature non-pregnant female mammals (except primates), is called oestrous cycle.

Monoestrus: The females which exhibit one oestrous cycle in a year is called monoestrus animals e.g., wild animals and bitches.

Polyoestrus: The females which exhibit regular oestrous cycle throughout the year, is called polyoestrus animals eg., cow, sow and doe.

Seasonally polyoestrus: The females which exhibit many oestrous cycles during a particular season, are called seasonally polyoestrus animals. eg., mare, ewe, buffalo and cat.

Proestrus: It is an ill-defined period during which the Graaffian follicles grow under the influence of FSH and produce increasing amounts of oestradiol.

Oestrus: It is the fairly well-defined period characterized by the intense sexual desire and acceptance of the male.

Metoestrus: It is a poorly defined period following estrus during which the corpus luteum grows rapidly from the granulosa cells of the ruptured follicle under the influence of LH.

Dioestrus: It is a longest phase of the oestrous cycle marked by mature corpus luteum.

Folliculogenesis: The process whereby immature follicles develop into more advanced follicles and become candidates for ovulation is referred to as folliculogenesis.

Anoestrus: Lack of oestrus expression at an expected time is called anoestrus.

Silent heat: A condition characterized by normal cyclical activity but without well-marked behavioural signs of heat or oestrus is called silent heat.

Pseudomenstruation: Several domestic animals shed blood from their uteri at certain phase of the oestrous cycle. This phenomenon is called pseudomenstruation.

Copulation or coitus: The insertion of erected penis into the vagina and subsequent ejaculation of semen is called copulation.

Calling : It is the term used to describe the vocalization of the queen (cat) when she is in heat.

Flagging: In case of stallion when intromission is achieved, ejaculation takes place over a period of a few minutes. During this time the tail of stallion is lifted up and down. This is called flagging.

Corpus haemorrhagicum: The blood-filled follicle devoid of the ovum is commonly called corpus haemorrhagicum.

Corpus luteum albicans : The degenerating avascular non-functional corpus is termed as corpus luteum albicans.

Yellow body : The mature corpus luteum (CL) of the cow contains a yellow lipochrome pigment which gives a light brown to yellow appearance. Because of this colouration, the CL is frequently referred to as the 'yellow body'. As the CL ages and begins degeneration, the colour darkens until it finally becomes deep orange to brown.

Dyspareunia: Painful or difficult coitus is called dyspareunia.

Induced ovulators : Animals that require copulation for ovulation are called as induced ovulators eg. cats, rabbits, ferrets, minks, camels, llamas and alpacas.

Oogenesis or Ovogenesis : Formation and development of the egg or ovum which begin from the embryonic stage and is completed when a spermatozoon penetrates the zona pellucida is called oogenesis OR Formation of ova from oogonia is called oogenesis.

Ovulation: The process whereby a secondary oocyte (Primary oocyte in bitch and mare) is released from the ovary following rupture of a mature Graaffian follicle and becomes available for fertilization is called ovulation.

Fertilization: The process of fusion of a sperm with a mature ovum is called fertilization. It begins with sperm-egg collision and ends with formation of mononucleated single cell (zygote).

Zona reaction: When sperm come in contact with zona pellucida, their head secrete acrosin (or zonalysin) enzymes which dissolve the zona pellucida and a sperm penetrates the zona pellucida. After entry of sperm to zona pellucida, some changes occur in the ovum which prevent entry of rest of the spermatozoa, called zona reaction.

Vitelline block: At the time of contact between sperm and vitelline membrane, a reaction occurs in the membrane, which makes it unresponsive to other sperm, called vitelline block.

Supernumerary sperm: The extra sperm which succeed in entering the vitelline membrane, inspite of both zona reaction and vitelline block are called supernumerary sperm.

Polyspermy: The condition in which more than one sperm get entry in the ovum, is called polyspermy.

Polygyny: The condition in which incomplete maturation of egg occurs due to failure to expel the second polar body resulting in a triploid zygote after fertilization is called polygyny.

Embryology: The study of the physiological development and growth of prenatal individual, is called embryology.

Implantation: The attachment of the conceptus to the tissues of the uterus, which commences at the blastocyst stage of development is called implantation.

Zona hatching: The process in which a blastocyst hatches or escapes from the zona pellucida in the uterus, is called zona hatching.

Intrauterine migration and spacing: Intrauterine migration and spacing of embryo or conceptus occurs in uterus for the survival of embryo in polytocous species.

Trophoblast or trophoectoderm: Differentiation of two distinct cell populations occur after blastocyst formation. The single peripheral layer of cells is termed as trophoblast or trophoectoderm. Later in development, the trophoblast forms chorion.

Embryoblast or inner cell mass: A group of cells residing at one pole beneath the trophoblast is called embryoblast or inner cell mass, which develops into three primary germ layers of embryo (ectoderm, mesoderm and endoderm) during the process of gastrulation.

Uterine milk or histotrophe: The uterine glands under the influence of oestrogen and progesterone secrete "uterine milk" which is composed of protein, fat and traces of glycogen, give nourishment to embryo.

Maternal recognition of pregnancy (MRP) : The critical period before the attachment of conceptus to the endometrium, trophoectoderm secretes a substance (interferon tau) which prolongs the life span of the cyclic corpus luteum beyond the period of the oestrous cycle. This phenomenon is called MRP.

Progesterone block: Under the influence of progesterone, the uterine endometrium releases very little $PGF_2\alpha$ and appears insensitive to oestrogen or oxytocin stimulation. This phenomena is called "Progesterone block".

Ovine trophoblast protein (oTP-1) or ovine interferon tau (oIFN): The ewe conceptus synthesizes and secretes an antiluteolytic product between days 12 and 21 of pregnancy called oTP-1 or oIFN- t.

Gestation or pregnancy: The condition of female characterized by presence of developing unborn young in the uterus is called pregnancy.

Gestation period: It is the period from fertilization to parturition.

Period of ovum or blastula: It is the period during which the conceptus sheds its zona pellucida and transforms to blastocyst. It is the period upto 10-12 days after fertilization in cows.

Period of embryo: It is the period between blastocyst and organogenesis. During this period, major tissues, organs and systems of the body are formed and changes in body shape occur so that by the end of this period, the species of the embryo is readily recognizable. It extends from 13ᵗʰ to 45ᵗʰ day of pregnancy in cow.

Period of foetus: It is the period during which most of the growth of placenta and foetus takes place and lasts until parturition.

Placenta: It is a fusion of foetal membranes to endometrium for physiological exchange.

Placentation: The process of formation of placental membranes around the foetus is called placentation.

Superfoecundation: The condition in which offspring from more than one sire are conceived at the same oestrus period, is called superfoecundation. Superfoecundation is observed more commonly in bitches because it resemble to ovulate two or more ova and have long heat periods. Therefore it has opportunity for mating by different males.

Superfoetation : Superfoetation occurs when an animal which is already pregnant comes into oestrus, is bred again and conceives a second litter. This condition is more common in multiparous animals eg., sow.

Telogony : It is the misconception that a pure bred animal mated accidentally by a mongrel may never breed true again. Believed occasionally by some dog & horse breeders.

Extrauterine pregnancy (or ectopic pregnancy): The fertilized ovum, embryo or foetus which establishes nutritive relations with organs or tissue **other than the endometrium** and undergoes some degree of embryological development is called ectopic pregnancy.

False etxrauterine pregnancy: An embryo or foetus develops normal placental relationship with the endometrium and the foetus reaches recognizable size. Thereafter, it escapes from the uterine cavity either into the abdominal cavity or the vagina, is called false extrauterine pregnancy.

Conception rate: Percentage of cows becoming pregnant after first service. It should be around 60% for chilled semen and 45-50% for frozen semen.

Number of services per conception: It is the average number of services required for one conception. It should be 1.5 services per conception.

Non-return rate: Number or percentage of cows not observed for oestrus after A.I.

Calving rate: Percentage of cows giving normal birth after first A.I.

Calving interval: The time interval between two successive calvings is called calving interval.

Service period: The period between calving to fertile oestrus is called service period.

Parity: It refers to the number of complete gestations (include the delivery of term or near term foetuses).

Placentome : It is the unit of close apposition of specialized area of endometrium (caruncle) with specialized area of the foetal membrane (cotyledon).

Pseudopregnancy: The condition in which a female has most signs of pregnancy but is not pregnant, is called pseudopregnancy. This condition is commonly found in bitch. The bitch comes in oestrus and is served but without fertilization or without development of any conceptus, she considers herself pregnant.

Pseudocyesis : The onset of lactation without parturition is called pseudocyesis. Generally, lactation without pregnancy in a bitch, is commonly referred to as pseudopregnancy by most of the owners and veterinary practioners. Actually pseudopregnancy is a misleading name for this because the bitch does not show signs of pregnancy but is only lactating.

Parturition: The process of giving birth to fully developed and viable offspring at the end of pregnancy, is called parturition.

Lochia: The normal uterine discharge during the first three-weeks after parturition, which consists of mucus, detritus and blood initially and later becomes serous, is called lochia.

Involution : The process by which the uterus returns to its non-pregnant size within specified time after parturition is known as involution of the uterus.

Puerperium: The period after completion of parturition during which the genital system is returning to its normal non-pregnant state is called puerperium.

Still-birth: Expulsion of dead foetus at the time of parturition, is called still-birth.

Premature birth: Expulsion of live foetus before completion of gestation period.

Abortion: The expulsion of dead foetus of recognizable size from the uterus before full term of gestation, is called abortion.

Vulva : The vulva is the external genitalia of female and consists of right and left labia. It is predominantly adipose tissue in which some fibres of the constrictor vulva muscle are embedded.

Clitoris : The clitoris in the female is the homologue of the penis in the male. It is situated just dorsal to the ventral commissure within the vulvar cleft.

Vestibule : The vestibule is the lumen of the **urogenital tract** between the vulvar cleft caudally and the hymen or transverse folds cranially or it is the tubular portion of the vulva connecting the labia with the vagina.

Vagina : The vagina is the muscular, tubular organ between the vestibule and cervix.

Vulvar cleft : The external opening of the vulva is called vulvar cleft.

Endometrium, myometrium and perimetrium : The tunicae mucosa, muscularis and serosa of the uterine wall are commonly called endometrium, myometrium and perimetrium.

Endosalpinx : The mucosa of the oviduct is called endosalpinx.

Middle uterine artery : It is a large branch of the internal iliac artery which supplies blood to most of the uterus.

Cervical Star: An irregular spot on the chorion found over the internal os of the cervix of mare, is called cervical star. It is constituted by **necrotic tips of the chorion** found at the apices of the chorioallantois.

Hippomanes: Amorphous, semisolid, amber-coloured, irregular shaped masses or bodies commonly found floating in the allontoic fluid are called hippomanes. Hippomanes are **allontoic calculi.**

Simple uterus : When a uterus has a pear-shaped body with no uterine horns, it is known as simple uterus. eg., woman's uterus and other primates.

Duplex uterus : When a uterus consists of two uterine horns each with a separate cervix, it is called duplex uterus. eg., rat, rabbit, guinea pig and other small animals.

Bicornuate uterus : When a uterus has a small uterine body and two long uterine horns, it is called bicornuate uterus eg., sow, bitch, cat, cow, ewe and doe.

Bipartite uterus : When a uterus has a prominent uterine body and two uterine horns that are not as long and distinct as in the bicornuate type, it is called bipartite uterus. eg., mare.

Teratology: The division of embryology and pathology dealing with abnormal development and malformation of the antenatal individual is called teratology.

Teratogens: The non-genetic anomalies or monsters are caused by a variety of environmental factors or agents. These agents are called teratogens.

Anomaly: If the malformation involves only an organ or part of the body, it is called an anomaly.

Monster: If the deformity or malformation is extensive, the animal is called monster.

Intersex: An individual having some of the characteristics of both the sexes and therefore showing abnormalities of sexual development, is called intersex.

Chimeras: A chimera is an individual composed of two or more types of cells, each type arising from a different source and containing different chromosome constitutions. This condition is called **chimerism.** Especially in livestock, a chimera containing cells derived from two **different zygotes.** This usually arises due to fusion between placentas during pregnancy and subsequent anastomosis of the foetal blood circulations. Free-martin is an example of chimera.

Mosaic: Mosaic is an individual consists of two genetically different cell types containing different chromosome constitutions but both derived from the **same zygote.** This condition is called **mosaicism.** A mosaic usually results from **mitotic non-disjunction** in a single zygote.

True hermaphrodite: An individual having both testis and ovary or ovotestes, is called true hermaphrodite.

Pseudohermaphrodite: An individual having gonads of only one sex (either ovary or testis) but external genitalia and secondary characters of opposite sex is called pseudohermaphrodite.

Male pseudohermaphrodite : An individual having **testes** but **phenotypically resembles to female,** is called male pseudohermaphrodite.

Female pseudohermaphrodite: An individual having **ovaries** but

335

phenotypically resembles to male, is called female pseudohermaphrodite.

Freemartin: (Free = sterile; martin = bovine) The infertile female with a modified genital tract born cot-win with a male foetus with which it has exchanged whole blood is called freemartin.

Twins: The two individuals that are born at the same time and from the same parents are called twins.

Monozygotic or identical twins: In this type, twins are derived from a single zygote that divides at an early stage of embryonic development. They are of the same sex and genetically identical.

Dizygotic or fraternal twins: In this type, twins are developed from separate zygotes during the same oestrous cycle.

Fused or Siamese twins: These are monozygotic twins which result from the incomplete division of a single embryo.

Schistosoma reflexus: The monster in which acute angulation of vertebral column takes place causing dorsal approximation of head and tail. The main defect is in skeleton. The thoracic and abdominal tunics are absent or incomplete ventrally exposing the visceral contents.

Perosomus elumbis: The monster in which vertebrae and spinal cord is absent after the thoracic region to tail. Therefore, the pelvis remains deformed, small and flattened and the hind limbs are strongly ankylosed and flexed. There is also muscular atrophy of lumbar and sacral regions with rigidity of joints.

Hydrocephalus: Hydrocephalus monster is characterized by swelling of cranium due to accumulation of fluid in the ventricular system (internal hydrocephalus) or between the duramater and brain (external hydrocephalus).

Polysarcia or lard claves: Polysarcia is the accumulation of excessive quantities of fat in the subcutaneous tissues.

Wryneck: A congenital deformity in which the head and neck are fixed in flexion due to ankylosis of the cervical vertebrae, arises during the peculiar bicornual gestation of solipeds.

White heifer disease: Due to arrested development of the Mullerian duct system, the uterus and the vagina are incompletely developed but the ovaries and vulva are always normal. This abnormality in heifer is called white heifer disease.

Eutocia: The safe, easy, natural or physiological parturition is called eutocia.

Dystocia: When the first or especially the second stage of parturition is markedly prolonged and becomes difficult or impossible for the dam to expel out the foetus without artificial aid, the condition is called dystocia.

Mutation: It is defined as those operations by which a foetus is returned to a normal presentation, position and posture by repulsion, rotation, version and adjustment of the extremities.

Repulsion (or retropulsion): Pushing of foetus out of the maternal pelvis or birth canal into the uterus, where space is available for correction of position or posture of the foetus and its extremities, is called repulsion.

Rotation: Turning of the foetus on its long axis to bring the foetus into a dorso-sacral position, is called rotation.

Version: Rotation of the foetus on its transverse axis into anterior or posterior presentation, is called version.

Extension and adjustment of the extremities: Correction of abnormal posture is called extension and adjustment of the extremities.

Force extraction: Pulling of the foetus through the birth canal by means of application of outside force or traction is called force extraction of foetus.

Foetotomy or embryotomy: It is defined as those operations performed on the foetus for the purpose of reducing its size by either its division or the removal of certain parts.

Caesarean section: Caesarean section is the delivery of the foetus, usually at parturition by laparohysterotomy.

Obturator paralysis: Injury to the obturator nerve generally observed after correction of hip lock in anterior presentation, characterized by the paralysis of adductor muscles of thigh.

Peroneal paralysis: Due to injury or trauma of peroneal nerve during struggle to rise (peroneal nerve passes over the dorsolateral condyle of tibia & fibula) resulting knuckling of the fetlock and dropping of the hock, and difficulty in rising, standing and walking.

Episiotomy: The technique to incise the vulva to increase its diameter for safe delivery.is called episiotomy.

Butt or Poll or Vertex posture: The downward displacement of head in which foetus nose is towards the trachea and the poll is presented at the pelvic inlet in anterior presentation and dorsosacral position is called vertex posture.

Nape posture (nape means back or hind part of neck): The downward displacement of head in which the head is flexed more than vertex posture so strongly that not only the poll but also the part of nape of neck is presented at the pelvic inlet in anterior presentation and dorso-sacral position is called nape posture.

True breast-head posture: The downward displacement of the head in which the entire head of the foetus gets dropped down between the fore limbs in anterior presentation and dorso-sacral position, is called true breast-head posture.

Foot-nape posture: The upward displacement of one or both expanded fore limbs so that the limbs come to lie above the extended head in the vagina in anterior presentation and dorso-sacral position, is called foot-nape posture. It is common in horse.

Breech presentation: The bilateral hip flexion i.e. both hind limbs are retained in the uterus in posterior presentation and lumbo-sacral position, is called 'breech presentation'.

Dog-sitting position: Anterior presentation with rear legs extended beneath the foetus called 'Dog-sitting' posture (Roberts).

- It is oblique ventro-vertical presentation in which the foetal head, neck and forelimbs are in the vagina accompanied by the distal extremities of both hindlimbs.
- This form of dystocia is seen very **occasionally in the mare and extremely rare in the cow.**
- Roberts considers that the dog-sitting posture is an abnormal posture of anterior presentation while almost all other authors (Arthur, Jackson, Benesh and Wright etc.) consider it as oblique ventro-vertical presentation.

Retention of placenta: The non-separation and failure of expulsion of foetal membranes within a certain time limit for particular species (for cow 8-12 hours), is called retention of placenta.

Uterine inertia: The lack of normal physiological uterine contraction during or after parturition is called uterine inertia.

Primary uterine inertia: The failure of the uterine muscles to contract normally at parturition due to hormonal imbalance, lack of receptor on muscles, diseases of muscles etc is called primary uterine inertia.

Secondary uterine inertia: The failure of the uterine muscles to contract due to exhaustion of the uterine muscles during prolonged dystocia, is called secondary uterine inertia.

Mummification: The process in which foetus dies within the uterus, autolysis occurs without putrefaction and the remaining shrivelled mass of bones gets enclosed by skin with persistency of corpus luteum is called mummification.

Maceration: The process in which a foetus dies after ossification within the uterus and the foetus undergoes microbial digestion or putrefaction in the fluid of uterus till only the mass of bones remains, is known as maceration.

Hydramnios: The accumulation of excess amniotic fluid in the amniotic cavity during the development of foetus is called hydramnios. This is often associated with inherited or acquired malformation of the foetus.

Hydrallantois: The accumulation of excess allantoic fluid in the allantoic cavity during the development of foetus, is called hydrallantois.

Foetal anasarca: The excess amounts of fluid in the tissue beneath the skin of foetus, is called foetal anasarca.

Uterine torsion: The twisting of the uterus on its long axis, is called uterine torsion.

Vagino-cervical prolapse: A condition in which outward displacement of vagina and cervix occurs through the vulva, is called vagino-cervical prolapse.

Uterine prolapse: The outward displacement of the uterus through the vagina and vulva is called uterine prolapse. It is also called **casting of 'wethers'** or **casting of the calf bed**.

Ovarian Cysts: are defined as follicle-like ovarian structures having 2.5 cm in diameter or larger and persist for 10 days or more in the absence of a corpus luteum.

Follicular cysts: are anovulatory follicles that persist on the ovary for 10 days or usually much longer, have a diameter greater than 2.5 cm. and are characterized by nymphomania.

Luteal cysts: are anovulatory follicles over 2.5 cm in diameter that are partially luteinized and persist for a prolonged period and are usually characterized by anoestrus.

Cystic corpora lutea: are non-pathogenic ovarian cysts which arise following ovulation.

Adrenal virilism: is characterized by a long standing cystic ovarian disease in which the cow becomes heavy and coarse, develops a thick neck and head and a steer-like appearance.

Paraovarian cyst: are found in broad ligament around the ovary and oviduct. These cysts are vestiges of the Mullerian duct system.

Hypoplasia of ovary: Failure of migration of primordial germ cells from the yolk sac to the developing gonad during embryonic stage is the cause of hypoplasia of ovary.

Repeat breeder: The repeat breeder is one that has normal or nearly normal oestrous cycles and oestrus period, and has been inseminated three or more times with semen from known fertile bull but fails to conceive.

True anoestrus: When the ovaries have no any structure like Graafian follicles or corpus luteum i.e. ovaries are smooth, then the condition is called true anoestrus.

Apparent anoestrus: When the ovaries have corpus luteum or Graafian follicles but show anoestrus, then the condition is called apparent anoestrus.

Embryonic mortality: When the death of conceptus occurs before the completion of embryonic period, it is called embryonic mortality.

Pneumovagina: Aspiration of air into the vagina, resulting in inflammation of the vagina and uterus and causes infertility.

Oophoritis or ovaritis: Inflammation of ovary is called oophoritis.

Salpingitis: Inflammation of fallopian tube is called salpingitis.

Endometritis: Inflammation of endometrium is called endometritis.

Metritis: Inflammation of whole thickness of the wall of uterus is called metritis.

Septic metritis or puerperal metritis: The metritis which occurs just after parturition i.e. within 1-10 days with systemic symptoms is called septic metritis.

Post-partum metritis: The metritis which occurs after 2 to 8 weeks or more after parturition, is called post-partum metritis. Here the animal does not show systemic symptoms.

Perimetritis: Inflammation of the serosa of uterus.

Parametritis: Inflammation of the uterine ligaments.

Sclerotic metritis: The complete destruction of endometrium as a result of severe chronic endometritis and replaced by fibrous tissue, is called sclerotic metritis.

Cervicitis: Inflammation of cervix.

Vaginitis: Inflammation of vagina.

Vulvitis: Inflammation of vulva.

Endometriosis: The old term "Chronic degenerative endometritis" is now replaced by endometriosis. Endometeriosis can be defined as a collective term to describe the wide range of degenerative changes like fibrosis and glandular degenerative changes.

Hydrosalpinx: The accumulation of fluid in fallopian tube is called hydrosalpinx.

Pyosalpinx: The accumulation of pus in fallopian tube is called pyosalpinx.

Hydrometra and mucometra: The accumulation of thin or viscid fluid in the uterus, is called Hydrometra or mucometra. Both hydrometra and mucometra are similar except for the degree of hydration of the mucin present in the uterus which may vary from a watery fluid to a semi solid mass.

Pyometra: Accumulation of pus in the uterus.

Metrorrhagia: Bleeding from genital tract is called metrorrhagia.

Embryo transfer technology (ETT): The technique by which fertilized embryos are collected from a donor female and transferred to recipient females that serve as surrogate mothers for the remaining period of pregnancy is called embryo transfer technology.

Superovulation: The artificial production of an abnormally large number of ova from an ovary is called superovulation. This is achieved by administration of FSH or eCG, which increases the number of follicles maturing and ovulating. OR superovulation can be defined as increased ovulatory response above a normal level by means of external hormonal therapy that would not be expected to occur naturally.

Synchronization of oestrus: Oestrus synchronization involves manipulation of the reproductive process by means of external hormonal therapy so that groups of females can be bred during a short predefined interval with normal fertility.

In vitro Fertilization (IVF): The fertilization of an oocyte by a spermatozoon outside the body of a living animal is called IVF. Oocytes obtained from living or recently slaughtered animals, are cultured to reach a certain stage of development before mixing with a culture capacitated spermatozoa.

PRID (Progesterone releasing intra-vaginal device): A stainless steel coil covered with an inert elastomer containing progesterone (1.55 gm) and oestrogen (10 mg) is kept in the vagina of a heifer or cow in order to influence the animal's oestrous cycle (oestrous synchronization).

CIDR (Controlled internal drug release device): A 'T' shaped device with flexible arms containing 1.9 gm of progesterone, is kept in the vagina of a heifer or cow in order to influence the animal's oestrous cycle (oestrous synchronization).

Transgenic animals : The animal in which a gene has been transferred during the embryonic stage through the genetic engineering is known as a transgenic animal.

Molecular farming : When the transgenic animals serve as bioreactors for the large-scale production of specific proteins; this approach has been popularly referred to as molecular farming.

Endocrine glands : The ductless glands of the body whose secretions go directly into the blood stream (which is in contrast to the exocrine glands whose secretions are carried away by means of duct) are called endocrine glands.

Hormone : A chemical produced by specific ductless endocrine organs which is transported by the blood vascular system and is able to affect distant target organs in low concentration is called hormone. However organs like the **uterus** and the **hypothalamus** produce hormones, which do not meet the criteria per classic definition of a hormone.

Base levels of hormones : Basel levels refer to a low and relatively constant level of the hormone in the blood.

Hormonal pulses : Pulses refer to a sharp and increased concentration of the hormone in the blood above the basal level of plasma concentration, lasting for short periods, **usually less than 1 hour.**

Hormonal surge : A surge is defined as a large, statistically significant increase in the concentration of a hormone in the blood above the basal level, lasting for more than 1 hour. The massive secretion of gonadotrophin particularly LH for a period, responsible for ovulation is called **LH surge.**

Episodic/tonic release : The episodic/tonic release of hormones (FSH and LH) means continuous basal secretion of gonadotrophin which stimulates the growth of both germinal and endocrine components of the ovary.

Growth factors : The hormones related substances controlling the growth and development of several organs, tissue and cultured cells are called growth factors. Unlike hormones, growth factors are produced and secreted by cells of different tissues (not specific endocrine glands) and diffuse into target cells.

Positive feedback mechanism : In this system, an increasing level of hormone (s) causes subsequent increase of another hormone. For example, increasing levels of oestrogen during the preovulatory phase triggers an abrupt release of LH.

Negative feedback mechanism : This system involves reciprocal inter-relationships between two or more glands and target organs.

Short-day breeder : An animal which starts to breed when the days are shortenining, is called short-day breeder eg., sheep.

Long-day breeder : An animal which starts to breed when the days are lengthening, is called long-day breeder eg., mare.

Pheromone : The chemical compound that allow communication among animals through the olfactory system are called pheromone or substances produced by an animal that act at a distance to produce hormonal, behavioural or other physiological changes in another animal of the same species have been called pheromone. In primates, including humans, pheromones also have effects. For example, women who are good friends or room-mates tend to synchronize their menstrual cycles. The armpit odour of women has been shown to be capable of modifying the menstrual cycle.

Sex pheromone : The pheromone by which sexual behaviour is affected is called sex pheromone.

Ram or boar effect : The exposure of ram or boar to the females advance the timing of the onset of puberty and is reffered to as ram or boar effect. This is mediated by pheromones which influence the

343

hypothalamic GnRH secretion.

Puberty : It is period when the endocrine and gametogenic functions of the gonads have first developed to the point where reproduction is possible. In the girls, the first event is **thelarche** the development of breast followed by **pubarche,** the development of axillary and pubic hair and then by **menarche,** the first **menstrual** period. Another event that occurs in humans at the time of puberty is an increase in the secretion of adrenal androgens. The onset of this increase is called **adrenarche.**

Precocious puberty : The appearance of appropriate secondry sexual characteristics before the age of eight in girls, is called precocious puberty. This occurrence is due to premature activation of intact hypothalamus – pituitary-ovarian axis.

Amenorrhoea : The absence of menstrual period is called amenorrhoea.

Primary amenorrhoea : When menstrual bleeding has never occurred, the condition is called primary amenorrhoea.

Secondary amenorrhoea : The cessation of cycles in a woman with previously normal menstrual period is called secondary amenorrhoea.

Hypomenorrhoea : When menstrual bleeding is scanty, the condition is called hypomenorrhoea.

Menorrhagia : When menstrual bleeding is abnormally more in quantity, the condition is called menorrhagia. **OR** when the duration of menstrual bleeding is prolonged or its quantity increased with unaltered normal cycle i.e. **4/28** becomes 7-10/28. The condition is called menorrhagia.

Oligomenorrhoea : The reduced frequency of menstrual period is called oligomenorrhoea.

Dysmenorrhea : The painful menstruation is called dysmenorrhea.

Delayed puberty : When puberty is delayed for as long as five years, it is called delayed puberty. The normal puberty and menarche have occasionally set in as late as twenty years in girls.

Menopause : The time at which menstruation ceases is called menopause. The meno pause occurs in women between the ages of 45 and 50, the average age is 47.

Precocious menopause : Menopause before the age of 40, is called precocious menopause.

Glossary

Climacteric : It is the phase of waning (declining) ovarian activity and may start two or three years before the menopause and continue for two to five years after it. The climacteric is thus a phase of adjustment between active and inactive ovarian function and may occupy several years of a woman's life.

Postmenopausal bleeding : Postmenopausal bleeding is any bleeding from the genital tract in a woman during postmenopausal age.

Abortion: Abortion in women is defined as expulsion of the foetus weighing under 500 gm. From 500 to 1000 gm, the infants considered *immature*, and infants expelled from 1000 to 2500 gm are called *premature*. The term miscarriage is often used, since the word 'abortion' is associated in the public mind with illegal procedures.

❊ ❊ ❊ ❊ ❊

Seeing much, suffering much, and studying much, are the three pillars of learning.

APPENDICES

Special Features :

- It is 'quick revision aids' which would certainly help the students during examinations, viva-voce and interviews without spending much of their precious time and energy in searching a lot of information in scattered form.

APPENDICES

HOMOLOGIES OF MALE AND FEMALE REPRODUCTIVE ORGANS.

Embryological structure	Adult female	Adult male
1. Gonads	• Ovary	• Testis
2. Mesenterium	• Mesovarium	• Mesorchium
3. Gabernaculum	• Round ligaments of the uterus • Proper ligament of the ovary	• Ligamentum testis
4. Paramesonephric duct (Mullerian duct)	• Oviducts • Uterus • Cervix • Vagina (cranial portion)	--Rudimentary
5. Mesonephric tubules	• Epoophoron* • Paroophoron*	• Efferent ducts
6. Mesonephric duct	Gartner's duct*	• Epididymis • Vas deferens • Seminal vesicle
7. Urogenital sinus	• Vestibule	• Penile urethra
8. Urogenital sinus	• Vestibular glands (Bartholin's glands)	Bulbourethral glands (Cowper's glands)
9. Urethral folds	• Labia minora	• Prepuce
10. Genital tubercle	• Clitoris	• Glans penis
11. Genital swellings	• Vulvar lips (labia majora)	• Scrotum

* Rudimentary

THE DIPLOID CHROMOSOME NUMBER OF DOMESTIC ANIMALS

Species	Chromosome number
Cattle	60
Water-buffalo	50
Swamp-buffalo	48
Horse	64
Donkey	62
Sheep	54
Goat	60
Dog	78
Cat	38
Camel	74
Fowl	78
Pig	38

THE ONSET OF PUBERTY IN DOMESTIC ANIMALS

Species	Onset of puberty
Exotic cow	8 to 18 months
Indigenous cow	24 to 30 months
Buffalo	24 to 48 months
Mare	18 to 24 months
Ewe	8 to 12 months
Doe	6 to 12 months
Sow	6 to 12 months
Bitch	6 to 12 months
Queen	5 to 12 months

DIFFERENCES BETWEEN UNIPAROUS AND MULTIPAROUS ANIMAL

Uniparous or Monotocous	Multiparous or Polytocous
• One ovum releases at ovulation	• 3 to 15 or more ova release at ovulation.
• Carry one foetus in the uterus.	• Carry more than one foetus in the uterus.
• Well-developed cervix.	• Poor-developed cervix.
• Placenta fills both the horns and body.	• Each placenta is limited to each horn.
• At the time of parturition the weight of foetus is about 10% the weight of the post partum dam.	• Each foetus is 1-3% of dam.
• Dystocia is common.	• Dystocia is rare.

LENGTH OF OESTROUS CYCLE IN DOMESTIC ANIMALS

Species	Length of oestrous cycle
Cow	21 days (18 to 24 days)
Buffalo	21 days
Mare	21 days (19 to 23 days)
Ewe	16.5 days (14 to 20 days)
Doe	20 days (15 to 24 days)
Sow	21 days (18 to 24 days)

LENGTH OF OESTROUS CYCLE OF PET AND LABORATORY ANIMALS

Species	Oestrous cycle
Cat	15 – 21 days
Bitch	6 – 7 months
Guinea pig	16 days
Hamster	4 days
Mouse	4 days
Rabbit	1 month

THE RELATIVE LENGTH OF VARIOUS PERIODS OF OESTROUS CYCLE IN DOMESTIC ANIMALS

Species	Proestrum	Oestrum	Metoestrum	Dioestrum
Cow	3 days	12 to 24 hours	3 to 5 days	13 days
Mare	3 days	4 to 7 days	3 to 5 days	6 to 10 days
Ewe	2 days	1 to 2 days	3 to 5 days	7 to 10 days
Sow	3 days	2 to 4 days	3 to 4 days	9 to 13 days
Bitch	9 days	9 days	--	--

APPROXIMATE TIME OF OVULATION FOR VARIOUS DOMESTIC ANIMALS

Species	Time of ovulation
Cow & Buffalo	12 to 14 hours after the end of oestrum, (heifer about 3 hours earlier than cow).
Mare	1 to 2 days before the end of oestrum.
Ewe	12 to 24 hours before the end of oestrum.
Doe	Towards the end of oestrum.
Sow	30-40 hours after the onset of oestrum.
Bitch	1-2 days after the onset of true oestrum.
Queen	About 27 hours after coitus.

351

NUMBER OF OVA PRODUCED BY DIFFERENT SPECIES

Species	Number of Ova
Cow & She buffalo	1
Mare	1
Ewe	1 - 2
Doe	1 - 3
Sow	6 to 20
Bitch	1 to 10 or even more
Queen	1 to 12

OPTIMUM TIME FOR SERVICE

Species	Optimum time for service
Cow	Just before the middle of oestrum to the end of the oestrum.
She-buffalo	5 to 8 hrs. before the cessation of heat or 16 to 20 hrs. after the onset of heat.
Mare	2nd-3rd day of oestrum.
Ewe	18-24 hours after the onset of oestrum.
Doe	24-36 hours after the onset of oestrum.
Sow	12-30 hours after the onset of oestrum.
Bitch	2-3 days after the onset of true oestrum or 10-14 days after the onset of proestrus bleeding.
Queen	During oestrum.

CHARACTERISTICS OF DIFFERENT GONADOTROPHINS HORMONES

Hormone	Mol. Wt. (Daltons)	Carbohydrate	Sialic acid	Half life
LH	28,000-34,000	12 - 24%	1 - 2%	30 minutes
FSH	32,000-37,000	25%	5%	2 hours
hCG	38,000	32%	8.5%	11 hours
PMSG	68,000	48%	10.5%	26 hours

TRANSPORT TIME OF OVA IN THE OVIDUCT AND ZONA HATCHING IN DIFFERENT ANIMALS

Species	Time in oviduct	Zona Hatching (After ovulation)
Sow	50 hrs (about 2 days)	6 days
Ewe	72 hrs (3 days)	7-8 days
Cow	90 hrs (about 3.5 days)	9-11 days
Doe	3 - 4 days	--
Mare	98 hrs (about 4 days)	8 days
Bitch	148 hrs (about 7 days)	11 - 12 days
Queen	4 - 8 days	11 - 12 days

EMBRYONIC DEVELOPMENT IN DIFFERENT ANIMALS (DAYS AFTER OVULATION)

Species	2-cell stage	4-cell stage	8-cell stage	Blastocyst	Zona hatching
Cattle	1 day	1.5 days	3 days	7-8 days	9-11 days
Horse	1 day	1.5 days	3 days	6 days	8 days
Sheep	1 day	1.3 days	1.5 days	6-7 days	7-8 days
Swine	0.6-0.8 day	1 day	2.5 days	5-6 days	6 days

DAYS OF MATERNAL RECOGNITION OF PREGNANCY (MRP) AND DAY OF DEFINITE ATTACHMENT :

Species	Day of MRP*	Day of definite attachment
Sow	12th day	18th day
Ewe	12th to 13th day	16th day
Cow	16th to 17th day	18th to 22nd day
Mare	14th to 16th day	36th to 38th day
Goat	17th day	--

CLASSIFICATION OF CHORIOALLANTOIC PLACENTAS :

Species	On the basis of		
	shape/villous pattern	Histological structure or maternal foetal barrier	Loss of maternal tissue at birth
Ruminant	Cotyledonary	Syndesmochorial	Nondeciduate
Mare and sow	Diffuse	Epitheliochorial	Nondeciduate
Dog & cat	Zonary	Endotheliochorial	Deciduate
Human and monkey	Discoidal	Haemochorial	Deciduate

ORIGIN AND FUNCTIONS OF FOETAL FLUIDS IN FARM ANIMALS

Fluid	Origin	Functions
Amniotic	- Foetal urine. - Secretions from respiratory tract and buccal cavity. - Maternal circulation.	- Protects foetus from external shock. - Prevents adhesion between foetal skin and amniotic membrane. - Assists in dilating cervix and lubricating birth passages during birth.
Allantoic	- Foetal urine - ecretory activity of allantoic membrane.	- Brings allantochorion into close apposition with endometrium during intial steps of attachment. - Stores foetal excretory products not readily transferred back to the mother. - Helps to maintain osmotic pressure of foetal plasma.

TYPE OF UTERUS IN DIFFERENT ANIMALS

Species	Uterus
Ruminants	Bicornuate
Sow	Bicornuate
Bitch	Bicornuate
Queen	Bicornuate
Mare	Bipartite
Women and other primates	Simple
Rat, rabbit, guinea pig and other small animals.	Duplex

GESTATION PERIOD IN DIFFERENT ANIMALS

Species	Gestation period	
	In days	In month
Hamster	15-18 days	--
Rat	21-30 days	--
Rabbit	30 – 35 days	--
Cat	60 days	2 months
Bitch	62 days	2 months 2 days
Ewe	145 days	5 days less in 5 months
Doe	155 days	5 months 5 days
Sow	114 days	3 months 3 weeks 3 days
Cow	279 days	9 months 9 days
Buffalo	310 days	10 months 10 days
Mare	341 days	11 months 11 days
Camel	410 days	1 year 1 month 1 week
Giraffe	--	14-15 months
Elephant	--	20-22 months
Tiger	105-113 days	--
Panther	90 – 93 days	--
Lion	108 days	--

STAGES OF GESTATION IN DOMESTIC ANIMALS

Species	Period of ovum	Period of embryo	Period of foetus
Cow	From fertilization to 10-12 days	From 13 days to 45 days	From 46 days to calving
Ewe	From fertilization to 10 days	From 11 days to 34 days	From 36 days to lambing
Mare	From fertilization to 11 days	From 12 days to 55-60 days	From 56 days to foaling

SIZE OF FOETUS AND GESTATION PERIOD IN CATTLE

Size of foetus	Gestational age
Mouse size	2 months
Rat size	3 months
Small cat size	4 months
Large cat size	5 months
Beagle dog size	6 months

CORRELATION OF FREMITUS AND GESTATION PERIOD IN CATTLE

Fremitus	Gestational age
Unilateral	120. days
Bilateral but asymmetrical	210. days
Bilateral and symmetrical	120. days (bicornual twins)

AVERAGE DURATION OF STAGES OF PARTURITION

Animal	Dilatation of cervix (first stage)	Expulsion of foetus (second stage)	Expulsion of foetal membranes. (third stage)
Cow & buffalo	2 – 6 hours	1/2 - 1 hour	6 – 12 hours
Ewe	2 – 6 hours	1/2 - 2 hours	1/2 - 8 hours
Mare	1 – 4 hours	12 – 30 min.	1 hour
Sow	2 – 12 hours	2.5 – 3 hours	1 – 4 hours

BIRTH WEIGHT OF DIFFERENT DOMESTIC ANIMALS

Species	Birth weight
Cattle	18 – 45 kg.
Horse	9 – 40 kg. (breed variation)
Sheep	4 – 5 kg.
Goat	3 – 5 kg.
Pig	1 – 1.5 kg.
Dog	100 – 300 gm.
Cat	100 gm.

STAGES OF PARTURITION AND RELATED EVENTS IN FARM ANIMALS

Stages of parturition	Mechanical forces	Period	Related events
First stage or dilatation of cervix	Regular uterine contractions	Beginning of uterine contraction until cervix is fully dilated and continuous with vagina.	• Maternal restlessness. • Elevated pulse and respiratory rates. • Relaxation and dilation of cervix. • Foetus adopt birth posture. • Chorioallantois enters into vagina (pseudo water bag).
Second stage or explulsion of foetus	Strong uterine and abdominal contractions	From complete cervical dilation to delivery of foetus	• Abdominal contraction starts. • Ferguson's reflex. • Maternal recumbency and straining. • Rupture of chorioallantois and escape of fluid from vulva. • Appearance of amniotic bag (true water bag). • Rupture of water bag and expulsion of foetus.
Third stage or expulsion of foetal membranes	Uterine contractions decrease in amplitude	After delivery of foetus to expulsion of foetal membranes.	• Loosening of placenta from endometrium. • Straining ceases. • Expulsion of foetal membranes.

Note : In polytocous species, second stage cannot be separated from the third stage.

TIME REQUIRED FOR INVOLUTION OF UTERUS IN DIFFERENT SPECIES.

Species	Time required
Cow	21 – 28 days
She-buffalo	21 days
Ewe	30 days
Mare	8 – 10 days
Sow	7 days
She-camel	10 days
Bitch	28 – 35 days

COMMON CAUSES OF ABORTION IN CATTLE :

Agents and common names	Incubation to abortion	Stage of gestation in which abortion occurs	Abortion rate
Brucella abortus Brucellosis or Bang's disease	2 weeks to 5 months or longer	6 to 9 months (Last trimester)	80% of unvaccinated cows infected in first or second trimester will abort
Campylobacter fetus ss venerealis	3 to 8 months	5 to 8 months	Usually less than 10%
Corynebacterium pyogenes	--	Usually in the last trimester	Sporadic or multiple upto 64%
Leptospira spp.	2 to 5 weeks after initial infection, may be 3 months	Usually in the last trimester	5 to 40%, may be sporadic or epidemic
Listeria spp.	May be very long because it appears to be stress related	Most in latter portions of last trimester (About 7th month of pregnancy)	Sporadic or multiple upto 50%
Salmonella		Anytime, 6 to 9 months	Usually sporadic but may be herd out-break.
Fungal Aspergillus spp. 60 to 80% Mucorales 10-15%	28 days after intravenous inoculation of spores, probably weeks or months after natural infection.	May be from 4 months gestation to term.	Sporadic to 5 to 10% of herd

Trichomonas foetus (Protozoa)	From breeding to any time upto 7 months	Usually in first half of gestation but may be upto 7 months	Very low.
Bovine viral diarrhea virus	4 days to 3 months after an outbreak	Usually early but may be upto 4 months	Usually very low but in uterine infection may cause severe intrauterine growth retardation in surviving foetus.
Infectious bovine rhino-tracheitis virus	2 weeks to 4 months	4 months to term	5 to 60%

CHARACTERISTICS OF GAMETES WITHIN THE FEMALE REPRODUCTIVE TRACT IN DOMESTIC ANIMALS

Species	Capacitation time (hours)	Retention of sperm fertility (hours)	Retention of ovum fertility (hours)
Cow	4	30-48	8-12
Mare	Unknown	70-140	6-8
Ewe	1.5	24	10-25
Sow	3-6	24-48	8-10
Bitch	7	150-240	>96
Queen	2-24	24-48	26

pH OF DIFFERENT PARTS OF FEMALE REPRODUCTIVE TRACT OF CATTLE

Part of reproductive tract	pH
Vagina	4.0
Cervical mucus	8.4
Uterus	7.8
Fallopian tubes (Follicular phase)	7.1-7.3
Fallopian tubes (Luteal phase)	7.5 – 7.8

COMPARISON BETWEEN THE OESTROUS CYCLE AND MENSTRUAL CYCLE

Events	Oestrous cycle	Menstrual cycle
Follicular phase	short (20% or less of cycle duration)	Long (50% of the cycle duration)
Ovulation	At the beginning and end of the cycle	Middle of cycle (day 14)
Luteal phase	80% of the cycle	50% of the cycle
Fertile period	24 hrs or less (5% of the cycle)	up to 6 days before ovulation (18% of cycle)
Endometrial sloughing	None	After luteolysis
Luteolysis	Uterine PGF$_{2\alpha}$	Ovarian PGF$_{2\alpha}$
Sexual receptivity	Well difined	Relatively uniform throughout cycle
Progesterone function and swexual receptivity	Inhibits GnRH release Inhibits sexual receptivity	Inhibits GnRH release Does not influence sexual receptivity

THE PLURAL AND LITERAL MEANING OF SOME IMPORTANT TERMS

Singular	Plural	Literal meaning
Ovary	Ovaries	Egg source
Follicle	Follicles	Little bag
Corpus haemorrhagicium	Corpora haemorrhagica	Body-blood clot
Corpus luteum	Corpora lutea	Yellow body
Corpus albicans	Corpora albicantia	White body
Oviduct	Oviducts	Egg tube
Infundibulum	Infundibulae	Funnel
Ampulla	Ampullae	Jug
Isthmus	Isthmi	Narrow part
Uterus	Uteri	Womb
Cervix	Cervices	Neck
Vagina	Vaginae	Sheath
Vestibule	Vestibules	Antechamber
Vulva	Vulvas	Lips
Clitoris	Clitori	-

❊ ❊ ❊ ❊ ❊

Good books are gold mines.

Index